CONTENTS

DEDICATION

This restored and revised reprint is, first and foremost, dedicated to its pseudonymous author at Sunræ Products Company, and second to my mother, Liselotte Erlanger Manfredi Glozer, my botanical mentor.

ACKNOWLEDGEMENTS

A book is never the work of just one person. I would like to thank my husband, nagasiva yronwode, and our colleagues Greywolf Townsend and Charles Porterfield for all of their help and support. Thanks also to Mary Hebda of the Ogema Public Library for research.

LET NATURE HELP YOU

Don't be in doubt about herbs. Know what each herb is used for and how to use it. Herbs have been employed for the relief of human ailments for many thousands of years and there are millions of people today who strongly believe in herbs and their cures. In this book there are over 350 different kinds of herbs, roots, and barks listed in alphabetical order, together with a description of what each herb is used for.

Sunræ Products Company
Ogema, Wisconsin

INTRODUCTION TO THE REVISED EDITION

Fifteen years ago i wrote a book called *Hoodoo Herb and Root Magic,* in which i detailed the basic information i had collected for the previous 40 years about how herbs, roots, minerals, and zoological curios are used in the practice of African-American folk magic. In that book i frequently made glancing references to the medical uses of herbs, but since medicine was not the focus of the text, i did not delve into the topic of how the conjure doctor has historically functioned as a *doctor*, nor did i remark at any length on the general American practices of herbal medicine as they were performed during my own youth by the two previous generations of practitioners who were my teachers in folk magic and the everyday skills of farming, gardening, animal husbandry, cooking, canning, sewing, spinning, weaving, quilting, embroidery, and midwifery.

WANT Profitable home work? Write Sunrae Products Co., Ogema, Wis.

This book — or, more properly, *This Amazing Book* by the Sunræ Products Company — is a glimpse at the other side of herbology, namely. the use of herbs in medicine. But there is more to it than that, and to explain why the preparation and revision of this little volume of herb-lore means so much to me, i should like to beg your indulgence for a slight digression

This Amazing Book takes me back to a different time in my own life, to the point at which i left urban society, never to return.

I had been a student of natural history and the arts and skills of basic human existence ever since i was exposed to the writings of Ernest Thompson Seton as a child, but it was only when i discovered the works of Gene Stratton Porter and Laura Ingalls Wilder that i came to realize, with a profound certainty, that i did not like the social structure of the era and place into which i had been born. As a teen, i poetically thought that i was "nostalgic for a past i had never known," or, to borrow a phrase from the comic books i loved, "trapped in a world i never made." However, all of those sentiments were wiped away in an instant when, in 1964, at Shimer college, i was exposed to the writings of John Locke, and learned the actual truth of my situation. My consent to be governed had not been sought — and, what's more, i did not consent to be governed!

This Amazing Book

Hoodoo Herb and Root Medicine

Opens the Door to Better Health

by

SUNRÆ PRODUCTS COMPANY

Illustrated by

F. SCHUYLER MATTHEWS

Restored, Revised, and Edited by

CATHERINE YRONWODE

Lucky Mojo Library of Occult Classics
Lucky Mojo Curio Company
Forestville, California
2017

This Amazing Book
Hoodoo Herb and Root Medicine
Opens the Door to Better Health
by Sunræ Products Company, revised and edited by catherine yronwode

Originally published circa 1947 as
This Amazing Book Herbs and Their Uses Opens the Door to Better Health

Text:
Sunræ Products Company [pseudonym], catherine yronwode, nagasiva yronwode

Editor:
catherine yronwode

Cover:
Greywolf Townsend, Josef Hanus

Art:
F. Schuyler Mathews
from *Field Book of American Wildflowers*. Knickerbocker Press, 1902,
New Edition Revised and Enlarged, G. P. Putnam's Sons, 1912.

Typesetting:
catherine yronwode, nagasiva yronwode

Production:
nagasiva yronwode

First Edition 2017

Published by
The Lucky Mojo Curio Company
6632 Covey Road
Forestville, California 95436
LuckyMojo.com

ISBN: 978-0-9961471-6-3

Printed in Canada.

In that moment, i was freed from my sentimental affection for the past and the precarious balancing act that it had imposed on my inherent political radicalism (love the Middle Ages, hate the monarchy; love the 19th century, hate slavery; love the Edwardian era, hate the lack of female suffrage; love the 1930s, hate the Nazis). I studied the anarchist writings of Josiah Warren and the sexual theories of Alice Bunker Stockham and Paschal Beverly Randolph and i became an active agent in the creation of my own life and lifestyle. I embarked on a conscious program of what later came to be known as "creative anachronism" — the willed ability to choose what i personally wanted from both the past and the present, and to use what i had selected to forge my own æsthetic and, most importantly, my own political path.

MAKE greaseless soap (five formulas) Herb Remedies (ten formulas) Good Money making tips (five). Everything 25c silver. Sunrae, Ogema 7, Wisconsin.

I immediately set about to learn, through hands-on practice, all of the historically vital skills and methods that i had earlier sentimentalized, while at the same time reducing the extent to which i interacted with agencies that could impose their laws on me, but would never be able to appropriate my consent. In common parlance, i became a hippie, of the subspecies known as a "back-to-the-lander" or "dirt hippie." Within a year my partner and i were living on an anti-war commune in eastern Washington state, gardening with horse and plow and reading by lamp and candle light.

FIVE Greaseless Soap Formulas, Ten Herb Formulas, Five Money Making Tips. Everything 25c. Sunrae, Ogema 7, Wisc.

For the next 15 years, at communes in California and Missouri, and through a second long partnership, i lived off the grid, far away from "televisionland," in happiness and sorrow, good times and bad, never thinking that i would return to the 20th century i had left behind. As a young mother, i supported myself by casting horoscopes; selling hand-made quilts, hand-spun yarn, hand-dipped candles, and herbal remedies; and writing about what i knew: gardening, sewing, and other "old-timey" skills.

The breakup of my second long-term relationship marked a devastating turning point in my life. Living way out in the country, i could not find another partner who shared my political or social viewpoint, and so my daughter and i drifted, half in and half out of a colliding clash of eras and lifestyles. Eventually i found work in the comic book industry, a profession that, in one form and another, i followed for 26 years. I settled on a compromise, a modern life with an urban man, whom i compelled to abide with me in a small, rural town. Eventually my daughter flew the nest, but i soldiered on, nose to the grindstone.

The end of that ill-suited union in the early 1990s allowed me to go back to writing about what i know and love. I became a staff editor at *Organic Gardening* magazine and i founded the Lucky Mojo Curio Company, a home business that is centered on the manufacture and supply of hand-made and herb-based folkloric spiritual supplies. I soon found a mate who is in tune with my æsthetics and philosophy, and although we live "on the grid," we happily still keep chickens, grow a garden, and maintain a model railroad; and with his help, i have been God-blessed to not have to enter the world of "televisionland" or subject myself to the grinding and soul-killing oppression of the military-industrial complex or daily highway driving or the fearsome National Football League.

One thing i have learned after all these years of creative anachronism is that few people are as eclectic as i am. When i wrote about organic gardening, few of my readers cared about comic books. When i wrote about blues music, few of my readers cared about quilting. When i wrote about sacred sex, few of my readers cared about model railroading. I have no intention to shove my enthusiasm for vintage restaurant ware china down the throat of those who seek me out to learn about spell-casting, but i do have one strong desire — to bring my friends from the world of folk magic, many of whom are urban, to a fuller understanding of what it is that they are actually looking at when they look at "conjure" or "hoodoo." They are not looking at "a system of magic" per se. They are looking at a *culture*, a culture in which magic walks hand-in-hand with gardening, cookery, sewing, and medicine.

Central to the development of this culture was the rural lifestyle. Both during slavery and after the Emancipation, hoodoo was primarily practiced among people who lived in the country. It was not until the First World War and the beginning of the Great Northern Migration that Black Americans began to leave the places where they had been born, fleeing from the Southern White culture that had deliberately held them back socially, financially, and legally. They left the countryside to seek their fortunes in urban centers like Chicago, Detroit, Dallas, Baltimore, Memphis, Houston, Atlanta, Saint Louis, Kansas City, Norfolk, Washington D.C., New York, and Philadelphia. As a result of the call for shipyard workers during World War Two, Los Angeles, San Francisco, and Oakland also became home to many recently-arrived Black families.

In the era of my youth, my Black school friends may have been born in California, but their parents and grandparents all seemed to hail from Mississippi, Texas, or Louisiana. This did not seem strange to me — after all, my mother had been born in Germany. We were the hopeful children of internal and external refugees, trying to build our own version of a fair and just society.

In listening to the older Black men and women who taught me hoodoo in the urban environment which they had only recently begun to inhabit, i learned all sorts of subsidiary skills, including how to keep chickens on the down low (don't have a rooster, only hens), how to make an herb tincture (use a brand of whiskey that represents what the herbs are for — Jack Daniels No. 7 for luck, Four Roses for love, Old Crow for death, Crown Royal for success, Johnnie Walker for health), and, above all, open your eyes, because the streets of the East Bay are lined with trees that bear edible fruits and only a fool would not pick and can them for the winter. Oh, yes, and if you can't find what you want locally, send for it from one of the order houses.

When i was young, herbal pharmacies and occult shops alike sent out beautiful and informative catalogues. These were called "order books" by most of my Southern-born friends. The Illinois Herb Company, Calumet Herbs, Indiana Botanical Garden, Nature's Herb Company, and others provided both medical and magical information about the herbs they sold. You could learn which roots were "carminative and stomachic" and which roots were "lucky curios" — and sometimes the same root functioned as both. The lines between medicine and magic were blurred, not only among the customers who used these herbs, but also among the dealers who supplied them. More than one medical herb company had a book department through which they offered esoteric and occult classics like *The Sixth and Seventh Books of Moses* and *The Secrets of the Psalms*. The same herb that "restored regularity to the bowels" might also "keep away evil," and the "reputed love herb" might do double-duty as a remedy for "all female complaints."

25 MONEY-Making tips 10c. Splendid possibilities. Sunrae, Ogema 7, Wisconsin.

The sense behind the dual usage of herbs for magic and herbs for medicine goes back to the earliest known writings about herbs. In the Classical era, when magic was not sequestered away as something "irrational" and medicine was not placed on a pedestal as unassailable "truth," people did the best they could with what they had. Not only poor people, but all people, used herbs for medicine and for magic.

I shall not bore you with the history of the Catholic Church and how it outlawed folk magic. I shall also not bore you with the history of how, by over-reaching the generally well-intentioned Pure Food and Drug Act of 1906 (which made the adulteration of pure herbal drugs illegal) a coalition of pharmaceutical company interests and the American Medical Association brought the entire field of herbal medicine to the brink of extinction. Suffice it to say that the refinement of plant matter into standard-strength white powders and pills — patentable, expensive white powders and pills — was deemed to be of enough economic value to lead inevitably to the outlawing of certain herbs (a ridiculous conceit!) and then to the levelling of threats of imprisonment against any herbalist bold enough to "practice medicine without a license."

The herb doctors did not go down without resistance. Joseph E. Meyer, known as "The Herbalist," made more than one impassioned and well-reasoned plea for freedom from governmental interference. He did not consent to be governed, and he resented it when, in the midst of his long and helpful career as an herb doctor, he was faced with legal threats against not only his own livelihood, but an entire way of life in which rural and small-town people provided for their own basic health care, using the well-known and well-understood active medicinal principles found in plants.

START Profitable mailorder business at home. Everything furnished. Details 10c. Suproco, Ogema, Wisconsin.

Well, all of that is gone now. The herb doctors lost. The term "doctor" was stripped from them, and only remains as a vestige among African-Americans, who still call conjure workers "root doctors."

Cut loose from its great and vital medical basis, hoodoo, especially as practiced in urban areas and among the young in the 21st century, functions primarily as a form of culture-centered magic. Because the 20th century institutionalization of racial segregation kept it under the radar of White authoritarian agencies, hoodoo did not disappear, but because root doctors and herb doctors of all races and cultures were hounded out of business, many practitioners of rootwork do not really know their roots, in either sense of the word.

START Profitable mailorder business at home. Everything furnished. Complete information 10c. Sunrae. Ogema. Wis.

So ... that brings us back to the Sunræ Products Company, also known as Suproco (SUnræ PROducts COmpany), and the reason i have set about to revise, restore, and edit this book.

All i know about Sunræ is contained in the short classified ads decorating these pages. They ran in *Popular Science Magazine* and *Popular Mechanics Magazine* from 1947 through 1949 and they are not much different than the many other such ads offering pickle recipes, handy farming tips, garden seeds, iris rhizomes, or treasured quilt patterns that one could find in the classified ads of *Grit* or *Farm and Dairy.*

The real contrast between Sunræ and other home businesses that took out similar classified ads was that Sunræ actually stocked and sold these hundreds of herbs by mail order for 50 cents per packet, and someone at the company wrote a wonderfully concise booklet on how to use them, had it carefully typeset by letterpress in tiny-tiny book format, and distributed it.

Here's what i have learned from the internet:

Ogema, Wisconsin is a town of less than 800 people. The word is Ojibway and means "a leader," specifically a wise, respected leader who has been selected by the general consent of the governed.

Nobody in Ogema seems to remember who owned and operated the Sunræ Products Company or Suproco. A Wisconsin city directory of the early 20th century shows that at least one commercial Ginseng grower was located in Ogema. Internal textual evidence points to the author being of German descent, because the entry for Caraway was originally listed as Kuemmel, its German name. And that's where the clues run out.

So, back to the text, because, for now, that is all we have.

STEADY Cash income by mail. Details 10c. Suproco, Ogema, Wisconsin.

The information contained in *This Amazing Book* is the same as that which virtually any herb doctor of the 19th or early 20th century would know. It is in agreement with such reputable sources as *J. M. Nickell's Botanical Ready Reference: Especially Designed for Druggists and Physicians* of 1881 and *King's American Dispensatory* of 1898, both of which were published before the virtual outlawing of herbal medicine.

Joseph E. Meyer's justly beloved *The Herbalist* of 1918 is the gold standard of popular books on the subject of medical herbalism, and might have been consulted. The prescriptions also generally accord with those given in Mrs. Maude Grieve's *A Modern Herbal*, published in 1931, a monumental two-volume compendium that embraces 2,000 years of herb doctoring, plus everything that modern chemistry had to offer at the time.

The author to whom Sunræ Products Company seems most indebted is J. M. Nickell, except that Sunræ retained an individualistic and local set of favoured common names for the medicinal herbs, and somehow managed to decompress Nickell's telegraphic style into readable English, presenting an amazing amount of useful information in a very small package.

In republishing this book, my husband and i have added the taxonomic binomials of the herbs (the "Latin names") and a series of alternative common names. He saw to the inclusion of 15 pages of beautiful illustrations by Ferdinand Schuyler Mathews from the 1902 and 1912 editions of the *Field Book of American Wildflowers,* while i expanded and revised a number of the entries and also added the guide to antique medical terminology, a few pages from my own lifetime collection of simple recipes for herbal medicines, and a one-page bibliography, to get you started on this path.

Despite the presence of a bibliography, people will ask me which books are best. I suggest that, in addition to the titles mentioned above, you also obtain *The Herbalist Almanac* by Clarence Meyer, *The Holistic Herbal* by David Hoffmann, and *Prescription for Herbal Healing* by Phyllis A. Balch.

What sets *This Amazing Book* apart from other herbals is that in this new edition we have keyed the medical herbs to their corresponding pages in *Hoodoo Herb and Root Magic*. When you see a notation such as "HHRM p. [0]" in a medical herb's entry, you may go to *Hoodoo Herb and Root Magic* and learn how that herb is employed in conjure. The notation "HHRM p. [0, *0*]," means that the second page number is an illustration.

I have loved this mysterious little volume for many years, and it is my pleasure and privilege to restore it, revise it, and present it to the conjure doctors of today, that you may find in it the rural roots of your rootwork.

— catherine yronwode

IMPORTANT NOTICE

According to the Bible, every plant was put on this Earth by God for the use of Mankind (Genesis 1:29). This book is published under the First Amendment to the United States Constitution, which grants us the right to discuss such matters of spiritual interest, and to express viewpoints that are not endorsed by the scientific community. The medical ascriptions of the plants given in this volume are authentic and traditional, and many attest to their efficacy — but please remember this: Although herbs and roots, when used in conjunction with prayer and other spiritual practices, have been known to work wonders, in some of life's gravest situations, your interests will best be served if, *before* undertaking self-healing, you also consult an appropriate professional such as a medical doctor, lawyer, social worker, minister, or the police.

Be aware, also, that some herbs mentioned in this text are poisonous or upsetting when ingested. Please use common sense. If a plant is noted as "purgative," "emetic," "cathartic," or "laxative" in these pages, do not chew it or drink it as a tea without a further study of herbal medicine. You could harm yourself. Likewise, some herbs can be irritating if applied directly to the skin, some may have ill effects if smoked, and even the most innocuous herb may cause dangerous allergic reactions in some people.

Many of these herbs are commonplace and can be found growing all over North America. Armed with a wild flower identification manual, you may be able to harvest them yourself, being aware of the fact that endangered or rare plants must not be disturbed. Others are common garden plants, readily propagated from seeds or cuttings, and you may enjoy growing them yourself. Some herbs are available in dry form, either cut-and-sifted or powdered, at grocery stores or health-food shops in most towns and cities. A few herbs are only carried by specialty supply stores and may be difficult to locate in your area.

If your local drug store cannot supply you with the herbs you need, we may be able to. We furnish many of the herbs in this book at the rate of six packages plus a free muslin tea steeping bag for $15.00 plus $5.00 dollars postage when you order the "Six Herb Tea Special." Clearly name the six herbs you require; we cannot prescribe for you. Allow two weeks for postal delivery. Our complete sales list is online and you can place orders at:

HerbMagic.com

A GUIDE TO MEDICAL TERMINOLOGY

Mid-20th century books such as this are both modern and old-fashioned at the same time. Excepting genetics, which had yet to come into focus as a cause of ill-health, there was a good understanding of diseases at the time that *This Amazing Book* was first published. Vitamins had been categorized, endocrinology was a growing area of research, and antibiotics had been introduced during World War Two. Still, many older lay people and herbal doctors continued to employ the medical terminology of their youths, that is, the lexicon of the late 19th century.

Time having moved on in the 70 years since *This Amazing Book* first appeared, i would like to begin by providing my younger and less antiquarian readers with a glossary of the medical words you will encounter in this book. Don't be alarmed, it is not overly long.

Some terms, like asthma and constipation, have remained unchanged over the years, but others, such as dyspepsia and gravel, are rarely used in the 21st century. This is not to say that the conditions no longer exist, merely that the terminology has changed. Dyspepsia is now called indigestion, heartburn, or gastric reflux, while gravel is now known as kidney stones. Additionally, older practitioners described diseases by their presentation or visible effect, not by their cause. Thus urinary suppression would be strangury, but the cause, whether cystitis, bladder stones, urethritis, prostatitis, or cancer, was undefined.

Changes in word usage are not the only reason i have added a glossary. Many people who want to use herbal medicines, and some who already do use them successfully, are unfamiliar with the body's systems, the names for what goes wrong in the body, or the causes of common diseases. By providing brief definitions of the terms used in *This Amazing Book*, i hope to encourage folks to learn about anatomy, to distinguish symptoms from diseases, and to gain self-empowerment and confidence when and if they talk to their primary care physicians, specialists, or pharmacists about their use of herbs as medicines.

Finally, a caution: *This Amazing Book* was written after the discovery of antibiotics, but the author chose not to delete diseases which might have been better treated with antibiotics, nor have i deleted any which might be better treated by the newer antiviral drugs. Please use good sense. Do not limit yourself to only herbal medicines if antibacterial or antiviral compounds will better serve you. The idea behind a life of creative anachronism is to select what suits you best from all of history, including today … and tomorrow.

- **Abscess:** A swelling in soft tissue filled with pus caused by an infection.
- **Affections:** Those things which affect or diminish the capacity of a bodily system. For example, pulmonary affections are disorders of the lungs; splenic affections are disorders of the spleen.
- **Agreeable:** A tonic or decoction which is of pleasant aroma or taste, generally distinguished from a bitter tonic.
- **Ague:** Malarial infection with paroxysmal stages of chills, fever, and sweating at regular intervals, followed by intermissions of varying duration.
- **Alterative:** Producing a salutary change without perceptible evacuation.
- **Anodyne:** Analgesic; an herb that reduces or eliminates sensations of pain.
- **Anthelmintic:** An herb that expels worms by stunning or killing them.
- **Aperient:** A very mild laxative that merely opens the bowels.
- **Asthma:** An inflammatory lung disease characterized by intermittent bronchial spasms, triggered by allergens and other environmental factors.
- **Astringent:** A substance that contracts or tightens organic tissues.
- **Bilious:** Disordered liver function and excessive secretion of bile with sensations of nausea, with or without vomiting; bilious fevers are malarial.
- **Bitters:** Tonics that taste bitter, typically by virtue of their containing medically active alkaloids, are collectively referred to as bitters.
- **Bowel Complaints:** This can refer to chronic constipation, chronic diarrhea, irritable bowel syndrome, gas, or even undiagnosed colon cancer.
- **Bright's disease:** Chronic inflammation of the kidneys; chronic nephritis.
- **Canker:** A herpes virus eruption. In the mouth, it is also called a cold sore or fever blister. Genital canker is genital herpes or human papilloma virus.
- **Carminative:** An herb that reduces the production of stomach gas or causes belching of stomach gas, preventing abdominal pain or flatulence.
- **Catarrh:** An excessive flow of mucus. Nasal catarrh is a cold, bronchial catarrh is bronchitis, urethral catarrh is gleet, vaginal catarrh is leucorrhea, suffocative catarrh is croup, epidemic catarrh is influenza.
- **Cathartic:** An herb or other substance that accelerates defecation.
- **Colic:** Abdominal pain and cramp; a disorder of the stomach or bowels that is attended with pain, also called gripes and bellyache.
- **Costive:** Affected with or showing a tendency toward constipation.
- **Cough:** A reflex of the lungs in which air is rapidly expelled to help clear the lungs of mucus, irritants, or microbes. It is a symptom, not a disease. Cough suppression treats the symptom.
- **Croup:** Obstructive laryngitis, a serious viral throat infection of childhood.

- **Cure:** A remedy that completely removes a disease, including its symptoms and the agent that caused it.
- **Debility:** Bodily weakness or feebleness; it is a symptom, not a disease.
- **Decoction:** A preparation made by boiling plant matter in water.
- **Demulcent:** A soothing substance that relieves irritation of the mucous membranes by forming a protective film.
- **Deobstruent:** An herb that acts to open the natural ducts in the body.
- **Diaphoretic:** An herb that induces almost imperceptible perspiration.
- **Diarrhea:** Frequent discharge from the bowels in a liquid form.
- **Digestive Fermentation:** The process by which food is broken down by microorganisms in the digestive tract for absorption into the bloodstream.
- **Diuretic:** An herb that rids the body of excess water and salt via the urine.
- **Dropsy:** Edema or swelling of soft tissues in any organ due to the increase or accumulation of excess water in the form of interstitial fluid.
- **Dysmenorrhea:** Painful menstruation; severe menstrual cramps.
- **Dyspepsia:** Impaired digestion, indigestion, heartburn, gastric reflux, belching, or upper abdominal fullness and pain after meals.
- **Dysphasia:** Impaired ability to speak, write, or comprehend language.
- **Emetic:** An herb, medicine, or other substance that causes vomiting.
- **Emmenagogue:** An herb that stimulates or increases menstrual flow.
- **Emollient:** A soothing moisturizer that makes the skin soft or supple.
- **Eruption:** Also known as eruptive disease; a localized inflammatory condition of the skin, including pimples, boils, eczema, and abscesses.
- **Erysipelas:** An acute, raised, red skin rash on the legs, toes, face, arms, or fingers; it is generally caused by infection with *Streptococcus* bacteria.
- **Expectorant:** An herb that increases the liquidity of mucus and lubricates the respiratory tract, aiding the expulsion of irritants from the lungs.
- **Felon:** A painfully infected abscess on the fingertip, also called a whitlow.
- **Female Complaints:** Pre-menstrual syndrome, dysmenorrhea, amenorrhea, endometriosis, adenomyosis, yeast infection, chlamydia, trichomoniasis, uterine fibroids, uterine cancer, cervical cancer, or ovarian cancer.
- **Fever:** Normal body temperature is 98.6 degrees Fahrenheit. Anything higher than 100 degrees is a fever. Intermittent fevers exhibit feverish periods alternating with periods of normal temperature, remittent fevers are those in which high and low fever alternate but the temperature is always above normal, and bilious or malarial fevers also include nausea and vomiting.
- **Flatulency:** Accumulation of intestinal gas and its expulsion via the anus.

- **Flooding:** Uterine hemorrhage in connection with childbirth or miscarriage; also excessive menstrual flow due to uterine fibroids.
- **Flux:** Dysentery, gastroenteritis, or diarrhea with blood, pain, and nausea. Bloody flux is a symptom caused by bacteria, viruses, worms, or protozoa.
- **Fomentation:** A warm, moist medicinal compress; an herbal poultice.
- **Galactagogue:** An herb that increases the flow of milk in a nursing mother.
- **Gallstones:** Bile, also called gall, is stored in the gallbladder until needed by the body. Solidified gall becomes gallstones. They may cause pain.
- **Gangrene:** Cell death caused by reduced blood supply to the affected tissues. It can be a life-threatening condition.
- **Gleet:** A watery discharge from the urethra caused by gonorrheal infection.
- **Gravel:** Kidney stones, also known as gravel, are solid pieces of material which form in the kidneys from minerals in urine; they are painful.
- **Gripes:** A pinching, spasmodic pain in the intestines; colic.
- **Hepatic Derangement:** A disease that impedes the function of the liver.
- **Herpetic:** Related to the herpes viruses: herpetic sciatica, postherpetic neuralgia, fever blisters, cold sores, canker sores, and genital herpes.
- **Hydrogogue:** A substance that induces watery evacuation of the bowels.
- **Hysterics:** A wild, exaggerated, overly emotional reaction to a stimulus.
- **Infection:** A disease caused a bacterium, fungus, virus, or protozoan.
- **Inflammatory Disease:** An inflammation or swelling.
- **Infusion:** A preparation made by steeping an herb in hot water.
- **Internal Lubricant:** A substance that relieves constipation without laxative action by providing a smooth, demulcent passage.
- **Jaundice:** A yellowing of the skin, generally linked to diseases of the liver and the bile tract, such as gallstones, hepatitis, or pancreatic cancer.
- **Laxative:** An herb or other substance that facilitates defecation.
- **Leucorrhea:** Mucous discharge from the vagina as the result of infection.
- **Lochia:** Postpartum vaginal discharge; contains blood, mucus, and tissue.
- **Malaria:** An infection by parasitic protozoa of the genus *Plasmodium*, transmitted by an insect bite. Also called ague, congestive fever, marsh fever, paroxysmal fever, and remittent fever.
- **Neuralgia:** Sharp intermittent pain along the course of a nerve pathway. Causes can be diabetes, multiple sclerosis, or infections, like shingles virus.
- **Nutritive:** An herb with value as a food; also, the nutrious value of a food.
- **Palpitations:** Disturbingly noticeable, hard, rapid, or irregular heartbeat due to agitation, exertion, or illness.

- **Parturition:** Childbirth. A parturient, also called a parturition accelerator, is an herb that speeds and increases the intensity of labour contractions.
- **Pectoral:** An herb that exerts a beneficial influence on the lungs.
- **Physic:** A medicine that purges; an herb that is cathartic or laxative.
- **Piles:** Inflamed or swollen hemorrhoids in the rectum.
- **Pleurisy:** A painful inflammation of the membranes around the lungs.
- **Poultice:** A soft, moist mass of herbs applied to the body to relieve soreness and inflammation; it is kept in place with a cloth; a fomentation.
- **Purifier of the Blood:** An herb that remediates blood-borne diseases.
- **Purgative:** Cleansing, especially by causing evacuation of the bowels
- **Remedy:** An agent that alleviates or remediates a diseased condition or brings relief from symptoms; it may or may not also constitute a cure.
- **Salt Rheum:** An eruptive skin disease; usually refers to eczema.
- **Scald-Head:** Any disease of the scalp with pustules, scales, or hair-loss.
- **Scorbutic:** Pertaining to scurvy, a disease resulting from a lack of vitamin C; an anti-scorbutic herb contains vitamin C and cures scurvy.
- **Scrofula:** A bacterial infection of the lymph nodes of the neck.
- **Sedative:** A medicine that reduces activity, excitement, or irritability.
- **Sialagogue:** An herb that increases the secretion of saliva.
- **Sick Headache:** A migraine headache with attendant nausea.
- **Soporific:** An herb that brings on sleep; a very mild sedative or narcotic.
- **Sore Mouth:** Mouth pain; generally speaking, herpes virus or cold sores.
- **Stimulant:** An herb that enhances alertness, wakefulness, and mobility.
- **Stomachic:** An herb that is strengthening and gives tone to the stomach.
- **Strangury:** Drop-by-drop urination; also called urinary suppression.
- **Styptic:** A substance that stops bleeding, also called a hemostatic agent.
- **Sudorific:** An herb that produces profuse perspiration.
- **Tetter:** A pustular skin disease; usually refers to eczema or ringworm.
- **Tincture:** A liquid extract made by soaking herbs in alcohol.
- **Tonic:** An herb that increases vigour or "tones up the system." A tonic is less stimulating, but generally easier on the body, than a stimulant.
- **Unguent:** A soothing ointment or salve spread on wounds, burns, rashes, or abrasions or used for lubrication of the skin.
- **Vermifuge:** An anthelmintic that stuns worms until they can be expelled.
- **Vesicant:** An herb or other substance that blisters the skin.
- **Vulnerary:** An herb used in the healing of wounds.
- **Water-Brash:** Dyspepsia with perceptible gastroesophageal reflux.

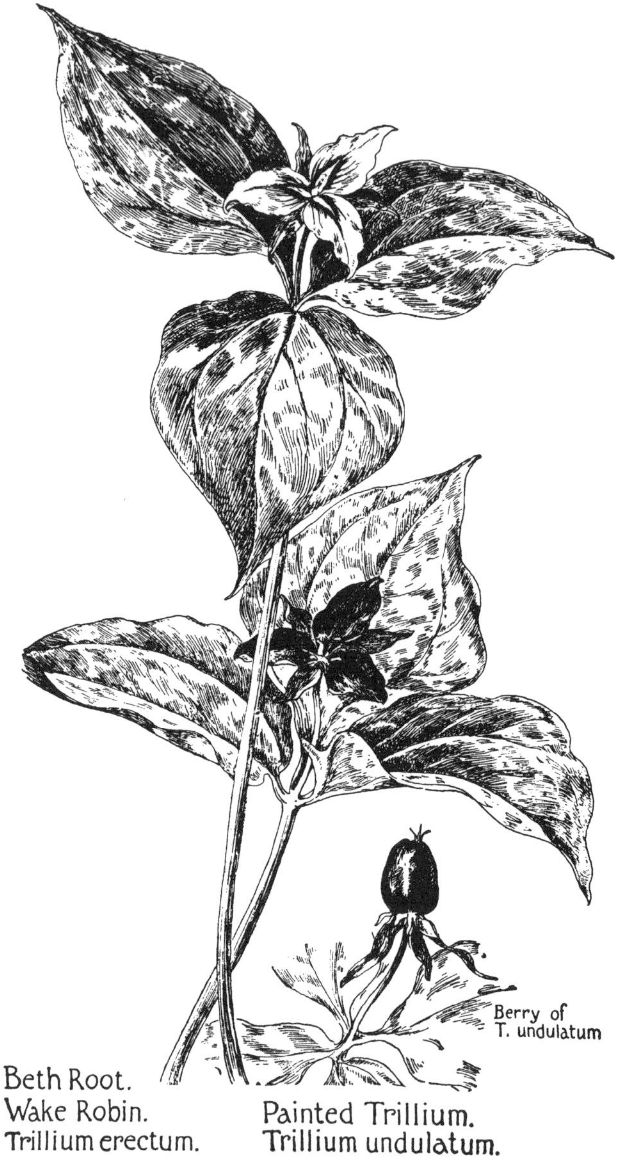

1. **Beth Root**, *page 24.*

ABSCESS ROOT **Polemoniaceæ**

(CREEPING JACOB'S LADDER, BLUE BELLS, SWEATROOT)

Polemonium reptans

Excellent for purifying the blood and for infections of the bladder and kidneys. Serviceable in pleurisy, fevers, inflammatory disease, scrofulous diseases, and in bowel complaints requiring an astringent, as an alterative, diaphoretic, and diuretic. Used topically for the bites of venomous snakes and insects, and as a gargle for bronchitis and laryngitis.

AGAR-AGAR **Algæ**

(CEYLON MOSS, SEA LETTUCE, SEA SPIRIT)

Euchema spinolum, Gelidium amansii, Gigartina speciosa, Gracilaria lichenoides, Sphærococcus euchema

Demulcent and internal lubricant. It has slight nutritive and culinary value as a natural vegetable gelatin or as a replacement for pectin, being agreeable to the taste and soothing to the digestion. HHRM p. 21.

AGRIMONY **Rosaceæ**

(COCKLEBURR, STICKLEWORT)

Agrimonia eupatoria, Agrimonia gryposepala

Highly recommended in bowel complaints, gravel, asthma, coughs. Said to be an excellent remedy for gallstones and to give tone and strength to the stomach. It is an astringent stomachic. HHRM p. 22, *23*.

ALDER, BLACK **Betulaceæ**

(COMMON ALDER, EUROPEAN ALDER)

Alnus glutinosa

Valuable as a tonic and purifier of the blood; used with excellent effect in jaundice, diarrhea, gangrene, and dyspepsia. A bitter astringent, the powdered bark is an ingredient in some herbal toothpastes. HHRM p. 24.

ALDER, TAG **Betulaceæ**

(HAZEL ALDER, SMOOTH ALDER)

Alnus serrulata

An excellent blood purifier and a gentle stimulant to the entire system; also valuable in scrofula and in all diseases of the skin. Tea made from the bark is used to treat diarrhea, coughs, toothaches, and sore mouth. HHRM p. 24.

ALFALFA **Leguminosæ (Fabaceæ)**

(LUCERNE)

Medicago sativa

This plant contains a large percentage of the enzymes or digestive ferments which aid digestion. The mineral content is the most important part, for it comprises all of the very important organic salts used in the construction and maintenance of the body, both animal and human. It is also especially rich in vitamins and iron, which are important in keeping the teeth firm and strong. HHRM p. 24, *23*.

ALTHÆA LEAF **Malvaceæ**

(HOLLYHOCK, MALLOW, MARSH MALLOW, ROSE OF SHARON)

Althœa officinalis, Althœa rosea, Althœa rosa-sinensis, Althœa zebrina, etc., also *Malva alcea* and many other *Malva spp.*

Emollient, demulcent, diuretic, pain-soothing, and lubricating; excellent in poultices and internally. See also Marshmallow Root. HHRM p. 28.

ANGELICA **Umbelliferæ**

(ARCHANGEL, DONG QUAI, HOLY GHOST ROOT, MASTERWORT)

Angelica archangelica, Angelica atropupurea, Angelica heterocarpa, Angelica officinalis, Angelica sinensis, Angelica sylvestris

A pleasant and agreeable tonic, very useful in cases of acid stomach, flatulent colic, heartburn, or water-brash and debility. HHRM p. 30.

ANGOSTURA **Rutaceæ**

Angostura alipes, Angostura trifoliata

Highly astringent and bitter; eases stomach cramps; useful in bilious diarrhea and dysentery, intermittent fever, and dropsy.

ANISE **Umbelliferæ**

Pimpinella anisum, Pimpinella major

Stimulant and carminative. Use in case of flatulency, colic in infants, and to remove nausea. Sometimes added to other medicines to improve their flavour, and as a replacement for Licorice. HHRM p. 31.

APPLE TREE BARK **Pomaceæ**

Malus malus

For intermittent, remittent, and bilious fevers, also gravel. Gives tone and strength to the system. HHRM p. 32.

ARBOR VITÆ **Cupressaceæ**

(THUJA, EASTERN WHITE-CEDAR, WESTERN CEDAR)

Thuja occidentalis, Thuja plicata

Expels worms and acts on kidneys and bladder, stimulating and toning up the system; the decoction is said to remove moles and moth-patch areas of discoloured skin, if persistently applied. Diaphoretic and anthelmintic.

ARNICA FLOWERS **Asteraceæ**

Arnica montana

Used topically as an anti-inflammatory in gout, dropsy, arthritis, and rheumatism; one of the best external applications for bruises and sprains. It should not be taken internally, as it can cause bleeding of the digestive tract.

ASH, BLACK **Oleaceæ**

Fraxinus nigra

Valuable as a remedy in eruptions and skin diseases; may be used as a wash in salt rheum, also when a tonic astringent influence is required.

ASH, PRICKLY **Rutaceæ**

(TOOTHACHE TREE, YELLOW WOOD, SUTERBERRY)

Xanthoxylum americanum, Zanthoxylum americanum

Stimulant, tonic, alterative, anodyne, and sialagogue. Used against colic and gallstones. A favourite remedy in chronic female troubles. Relieves toothache.

ASH, WAFER **Rutaceæ**

(HOPTREE, PICKAWAY ANISE, PTELIA, STINKING ASH, STINKING PRAIRIE BUSH, AGUE BARK)

Ptelea trifoliata

Much employed as a blood purifier, also as a vermifuge; it is highly recommended in intermittent and remittent fever, asthma, pulmonary affections, indigestion, and dysphasia. The seeds can be used as a substitution for Hops in beer-making.

ASH, WHITE **Oleaceæ**

(COMMON ASH, WEEPING ASH, WHITE ASH)

Fraxinus americana, Fraxinus excelsior

A mild diuretic and a cathartic laxative, useful in constipation, in dropsy, and urinary troubles, and also taken to reduce fat and weight. A poultice of the leaves is effective when applied to insect bites. HHRM p. 34.

BALM OF GILEAD BUDS

(TRUE BALM OF GILEAD) **Burseraceæ**

Commiphora opobalsamum, Commiphora gileadens

(BALM OF GILEAD, BALSAM POPLAR) **Salicaceæ**

Populus balsamifera, Populus candicans, Populus gileadensis, Populus tacomahaca

(BALM OF GILEAD, CANADA BALSAM, BALSAM FIR) **Pinaceæ**

Abies balsamea

Soaked in alcohol, an excellent application for cuts and bruises. Steeped in unsalted butter, olive oil, or tallow will give a most healing salve or unguent. Valuable as a decoction in coughs, colds, and lung trouble, also kidney and urinary difficulties. HHRM p. 35.

BALM, SWEET **Labiatæ**

(BALM, BEE BALM, LEMON BALM, LEMON MINT, SWEET MELISSA)

Melissa officinalis, Mentha citrata, Nepeta citriodora

Valuable in cases of flatulence, nausea, and vomiting attendant upon sick headache, and helpful to assist in menstruation or as a regulator in female complaints and female periodic headache. Useful in settling the stomach generally; also very useful in cases of low fever, and for kidney and bladder troubles, such as suppression of urine. HHRM p. 123.

BALMONY **Plantaginaceæ (Scrophulariaceæ, Veronicaceæ)**

(SNAKE HEAD, TURTLE HEAD, SALT RHEUM WEED)

Chelone glabra

A bitter anti-bilious tonic, mild laxative, and blood purifier; especially valuable in cases of jaundice and liver troubles; it also excites the digestive organs. Equally valuable as an anthelmintic to remove worms in children, either as a tea or in the form of an enema. As an ointment it is recommended for salt rheum, tetter, and piles. HHRM p. 187, *171*.

BARBERRY **Berberidaceæ**

(HOLY THORN, MAHONIA, MOUNTAIN GRAPE, OREGON GRAPE)

Berberis aquifolium, Berberis asiatica, Berberis vulgaris, Mahonia aquifolium

An excellent all-around tonic for general debility, producing a sense of vigour. Effective in severe cases of liver troubles and jaundice, as a laxative, alterative, antiseptic, and tonic. It makes an excellent gargle for a sore mouth. The berries possess astringent and anti-scorbutic properties. HHRM p. 37.

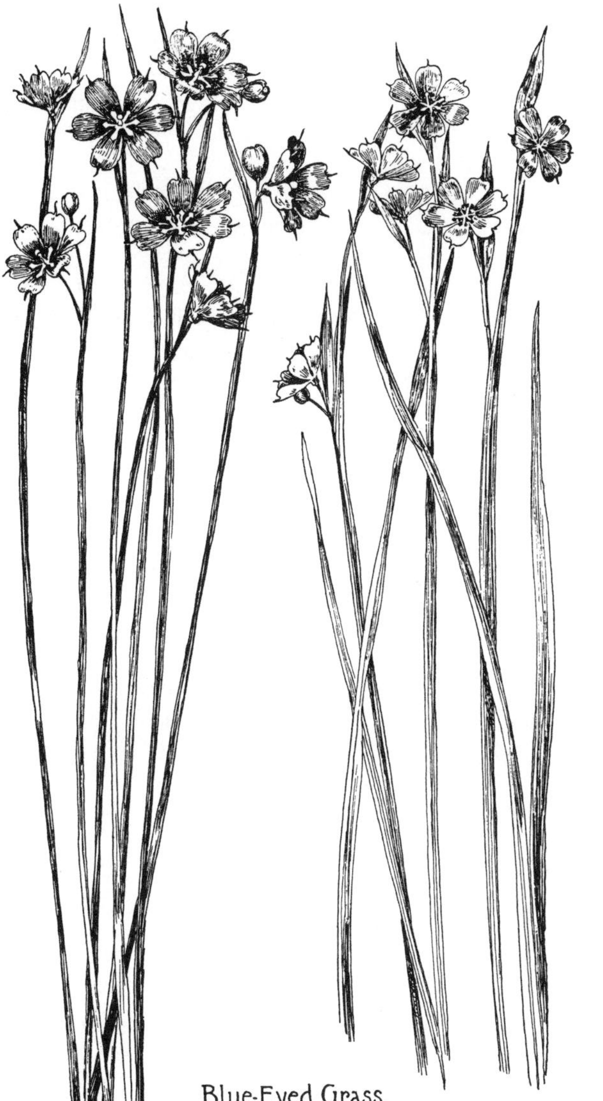

2. **Blue-Eyed Grass**, *page 26.*

BASIL **Labiatæ**

(HOLY BASIL, SACRED BASIL, SWEET BASIL, TULSI)

Ocimum basilicum, other Ocimum spp.

Recommended to allay excessive vomiting. It is a warm and grateful tonic and stimulant. Has well-known culinary uses. HHRM p. 37.

BAY **Lauraceæ**

(BAY LAUREL, BAY LEAF, GRECIAN BAY, LAUREL, SWEET BAY)

Laurus nobilis

A pleasant tonic, giving tone and strength to the digestive organs. Highly useful for expelling wind from the stomach and bowels, and excellent as an astringent. Much used for the flavouring of stews; it is also a useful and popular ingredient in both hair tonics and perfumes. HHRM p. 38.

BAYBERRY BARK **Myricaceæ**

(CANDLE BERRY, TALLOW SHRUB, WAX BERRY, WAX MYRTLE)

Pimenta acris, Myrica cerifera, Myrica gale, Myrica pennsylvanica

Valuable in diarrhea, jaundice, scrofula, canker in the mouth, and as a wash for spongy gums. Powdered as a snuff for catarrh. HHRM p. 39.

BEECH DROPS **Orobanchaceæ**

Epifagus virginiana, Orobanche uniflora

An eminent astringent. Used with benefit in fluxes and diarrhea. In erysipelas, the tea is ingested and the parts are also bathed with it. The decoction made into a poultice helps both fresh and old wounds to heal.

BEECH LEAVES **Fagaceæ**

Fagus sylvatica, Fagus grandifolia, Fagus crenata, Fagus lucida

Very useful in diabetes, cutaneous diseases, ulcers, and dyspepsia; also soothing, softening and healing to wounds. A good tonic and appetizer.

BETH ROOT **Liliaceæ**

(TRILLIUM, WAKE-ROBIN, BIRTH ROOT, RATTLESNAKE ROOT, DIXIE JOHN ROOT, SOUTHERN JOHN THE CONQUEROR)

Trillium erectum, Trillium pendulum, Trillium pendulatum

Astringent and tonic expectorant; most valuable in coughs, asthma, hectic fever, bloody urine, and derangement of the female generative organs. Recommended to promote parturition and reduce flooding. As a poultice, it is applied to bruises and piles. *Illustration: p. 18.* HHRM p. 189.

BETONY **Labiatæ**

(WOOD BETONY, LOUSEWORT)

Betonica officinalis, Pedicularis canadensis, Stachys betonica

For headaches, hysterics, palpitations, and extreme nervousness; quieting and easing to pain, neuralgia, and all nervous affections. HHRM p. 207, *197.*

BILBERRY **Vacciniaceæ**

(HUCKLEBERRY, BLACK WHORTLEBERRY, BLUE WHORTLEBERRY, SQUAW HUCKLEBERRY, WHORTLEBERRY)

Vaccinium myrtillus, Vaccinium frondosum, Vaccinium resinosum

Astringent, anti-scorbutic. Valuable in diarrhea and diabetes. HHRM p. 114.

BIRCH, SWEET **Betulaceæ**

(WHITE BIRCH)

Betula alba, Betula benta, Betula papyracea

Used with excellent effect in diarrhea or dysentery, to give tone to the bowels after exhausting discharges. The tea is aromatic, anti-rheumatic, stimulant, diaphoretic, and astringent. As a decoction or syrup it is useful in gravel and female obstructions.

BISTORT **Polygonaceæ**

(SNAKE WEED, RED LEGS, PATIENCE DOCK)

Polygonum bistorta

Use in diarrhea or whenever a general tonic astringent is needed; acts also on kidneys, increasing the flow of urine. HHRM p. 188.

BITTER ROOT **Apocynaceæ**

(DOGBANE, MILKWEED ROOT, SPREADING DOGBANE)

Apocynum androsæmifolium

Acts on the bowels and kidneys; is useful in expelling worms. Valuable in chronic liver complaints such as the ascites of hepatic cirrhosis. Helpful in dropsy due to heart failure, if dosage is closely monitored. HHRM p. 87.

BITTERSWEET TWIGS **Celastracaceæ**

(AMERICAN BITTERSWEET, CLIMBING BITTERSWEET)

Celastrus scandens

Employed in cutaneous diseases, scrofula, jaundice, and rheumatic complaints. The berries are poison, not to be taken as tea, but when steeped in pure lard or other unguent, the twigs make an excellent skin salve. HHRM p. 48, *23.*

BLACKBERRY ROOT **Rosaceæ**

(BRAMBLE, BRAMBLEBERRY)

Rubus fruticosus, Rubus villosus

A favourite and valuable remedy for cholera infantum, diarrhea, dysentery, and relaxed condition of intestines in children. HHRM p. 49.

BLACK COHOSH ROOT **Ranunculaceæ**

(BLACK SNAKE ROOT, BUGBANE, RATTLESNAKE ROOT)

Cimicifuga racemosa, Cimicifuga serpentaria

Much used in rheumatism, dropsy, epilepsy, and spasmodic affections. Valued in female complaints and as a parturition accelerator. HHRM p. 54. *47.*

BLACK ROOT **Scrophulariaceæ**

(BEAUMONT ROOT, BLACK MASTER, CULVER'S PHYSIC, CULVER'S ROOT, LEPTANDRA, PHYSIC ROOT)

Leptandra virginica, Eustachya purpurea, Pæderota virginica, Veronica virginica

For constipation and indigestion; a valuable tonic in cases of typhoid fever. Excellent in bilious and liver complaints; removes bile from the system. If too great a dose is taken, it can be cathartic and emetic. HHRM p. 53.

BLOOD ROOT **Papaveraceæ**

(COON ROOT, PUCCOON ROOT, RED PUCCOON, RED PAINT ROOT, TETTERWORT)

Sanguinaria canadensis, Sanguinaria minor

A useful remedy for coughs, colds, bronchitis, pneumonia, catarrh, and all affections of the respiratory organs; also valuable in typhoid, scarlatina, jaundice, dyspepsia, and, as a salve for ringworm. HHRM p. 55, *47.*

BLUE COHOSH **Berberidaceæ**

(PAPOOSE ROOT)

Caulophyllum thalictroides

Emmenagogue, parturient, and anti-spasmodic; employed in cramps, uterine inflammations, colic, hiccoughs, epilepsy, and hysteria. HHRM p. 55, *21.*

BLUE-EYED GRASS **Iridaceæ**

(BLUE-EYED FLOWERS)

Sisyrinchium angustifolium

Demulcent and emollient. A tea of the root treats diarrhea in children; a tea of the whole plant treats worms and stomach ache. *Illustration: p. 23.*

BLUE FLAG ROOT **Iridaceæ**

(WATER FLAG, SNAKE LILY)

Iris versicolor

A valuable alterative, cathartic, sialagogue, and diuretic. It stimulates the liver and is used in constipation and biliousness. *Illustration: p. 28.* HHRM p. 56.

BLUE VERVAIN **Verbenaceæ**

(AMERICAN VERBENA, SWAMP VERBENA)

Verbena hastata

Tonic, expectorant, sudorific, and anti-spasmodic. Aids poor circulation, corrects diseases of the stomach, helps coughs and liver complaints, and also a good galactagogue. Used as a poultice for piles.

BOLDO **Monimiaceæ**

Boldoa fragrans, Peumus boldoa, Peumus boldus

Antiseptic, tonic. Used in dyspepsia, catarrh of the bladder, and genito-urinary inflammation. It can be toxic if ingested. HHRM p. 57.

BONESET **Compositæ**

(THOROUGHWORT, WHITE SNAKE ROOT)

Eupatorium perfoliatum, Eupatorium rugosum, Eupatorium urticæfolium

A most valuable remedy for breaking up colds and fevers; also efficient for dyspepsia, jaundice, ague, and general debility of the system. HHRM p. 57, 2.

BORAGE **Boraginaceæ**

Borago officinalis

Diaphoretic; the honey-sweetened infusion eases sore throat. HHRM p. 57.

BRIER HIPS **Rosaceæ**

(SWEETBRIAR)

Rosa rubiginosa

Anti-scorbutic. Helps with kidney gravel. *Illustration: p. 33.* HHRM p. 168.

BROOM TOPS **Leguminosæ**

(GENISTA, GREEN BROOM, IRISH BROOM, SCOTCH BROOM)

Cytisus scoparius, Genista scoparius

Diuretic for kidney and bladder troubles; especially beneficial in dropsy. Combined with Uva-Ursi and Cleavers, always increases the flow of urine.

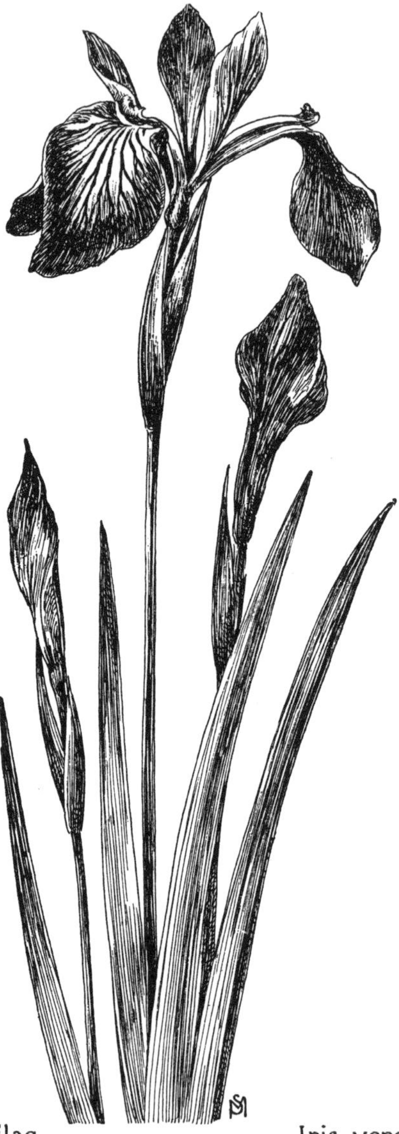

Blue Flag. Iris versicolor.

3. **Blue Flag**, *page 27.*

BRYONY **Cucurbitaceæ**

(RED BRYONY, WHITE BRYONY, WILD NEP, WILD VINE)

Bryonia alba, Bryonia dioica

A powerfully active and irritative hydragogue cathartic, producing watery discharges. Its action is similar to, but less predictable than, Jalap. Its use as a purgative is considered dangerous.

BUCHU **Rutaceæ**

Agathosma betulina, Agathosma crenulata, Barosma betulina, Barosma crenulata, Barosma serratifolia, Diosma crenulata, Diosma ericoides

Very useful in derangements of the urinary organs; one of the best known remedies to soothe the irritation of these organs. Used with excellent results for catarrh of the bladder and in cases of pain in urinating. HHRM p. 59.

BUCKBEAN **Gentianaceæ**

(BOGBEAN, WATER TREFOIL, MARSH CLOVER)

Menyanthes trifoliata

Acts on kidneys and bowels, expels worms, and is accounted an excellent remedy for catarrh of the stomach, dyspepsia, scurvy, and rheumatism.

BUCKHORN BRAKE **Osmundaceæ**

(FLOWERING FERN, LADY BRAKE, ROYAL FERN)

Osmunda cinnamomea, Osmunda regalis, Osmunda spectabilis

Very valuable in female weakness, cough, and dysentery. HHRM p. 93.

BUCKTHORN **Ramnaceæ**

(FRANGULA BARK, HIGHWAYTHORN, RAMSTHORN)

Rhamnus cathartica, Rhamnus frangula

One of the most effective laxative remedies known for chronic costiveness, serving to keep the bowels regular. It is also used in cases of gout, rheumatism, dropsy, and eruptive diseases, to clear the skin. Similar in effect to Cascara Sagrada. HHRM p. 65.

BUGLE WEED **Labiatæ**

(SWEET BUGLE, WATER BUGLE)

Lycopus virginicus

Sedative, astringent, and soporific. Produces gentle sleep, very useful in intermittent fever and hemorrhage of the lungs, bowels, and stomach. Valuable also in diabetes and useful in a compound for Bright's disease.

BURDOCK **Compositæ**

(BATWEED, BEGGAR'S BUTTONS, THORNY BURR)

Arctium lappa, Arctium minum

The root is one of the very best blood purifiers, used in scorbutic and scrofulous diseases, eliminating very rapidly any impurity or poison from the blood. It is also used in gout. HHRM p. 61, *47.*

BUTTERNUT BARK **Juglandaceæ**

(WHITE WALNUT, OILNUT)

Juglans cinerea

Used in habitual constipation as a gentle and agreeable laxative, acting on the liver. It has been employed as a mild vermifuge, suitable for children.

BUTTON SNAKE ROOT **Compositæ**

(BLAZING STAR, DEVIL'S BIT, GAY FEATHER, LIATRIS, RATTLESNAKE CONQUEROR, RATTLESNAKE MASTER)

Liatris scariosa, Liatris squarrosa, Liatris spicata

Valuable in scrofula, menstrual irregularity, and gleet. A gargle made from the tea is efficacious for sore throat. As a diuretic it is also used in Bright's disease when combined with Bugle Weed. HHRM p. 62, *71.*

CANADA SNAKE ROOT **Aristolochiaceæ**

(AMERICAN GINGER, CANADIAN GINGER, INDIAN GINGER, SNAKE ROOT GINGER, WILD GINGER)

Asarum canadense, Asarum virginicum

An agreeable carminative remedy for wind colic when taken as tea. It is also diaphoretic and sudorific, depending upon the dosage, and reliably eases perspiration. As a sialagogue it promotes both digestive salivation and expectoration as an aid to clearing the throat and lungs. It is, finally, a moderate diuretic of use in cases of dropsy. HHRM p. 102.

CANCER ROOT **Orobanchaceæ**

(AMERICAN CANCER ROOT)

Conopholis americana, Conopholis alpina

Very beneficial in cases of diarrhea, hemorrhage of the bowels and uterus, and for internal ulcers. Also valuable in erysipelas and as a local application to arrest the tendency of ulcers and wounds to gangrene. The name does not refer to it being a curative for cancer; rather, that it is a parasitic plant.

CARAWAY **Umbelliferæ**

(KUEMMEL)

Carum carvi

Used to relieve flatulent colic in infants, as a corrective to improve the flavour of disagreeable medicines, and also as a pleasant cooking and baking spice. It is carminative, stimulant, diuretic, and stomachic. HHRM p. 64.

CARDAMOM **Zingiberaceæ**

Alpinia cardamomum, Amomum cardamomum, Elettaria cardamomum

A warm and grateful aromatic used to prevent indigestion, remedy flatulence, and as a flavour corrective for bitter herbal medicines. It has culinary uses and is also added to teas to flavour them. HHRM p. 65.

CARROT, WILD **Apiaceæ**

(BIRD'S NEST, BEES' NEST, QUEEN ANNE'S LACE)

Daucus carota, Daucus pusillus

Diuretic, stimulant; useful for kidney and bladder trouble, dropsy, gravel, and strangury, and as a poultice in foul open sores. *Illustration: p. 38.*

CASCARA SAGRADA **Ramnaceæ**

(BUCKTHORN, CALIFORNIA BUCKTHORN, SACRED BARK)

Rhamnus purshiana

Its exclusive use is that of a laxative, and it is one of the best, as well as an excellent general intestinal tonic. Its continued use is beneficial in cases of gallstones and in chronic constipation. Similar to Buckthorn. HHRM p. 65.

CASCARILLA **Euphorbiaceæ**

(SWEETWOOD BARK, SWEET BARK, BAHAMA CASCARILLA)

Croton eleuteria

An aromatic, bitter tonic and stimulant, useful in dyspepsia, water-brash, and flatulence. In chronic bronchitis it is used as an expectorant.

CATNIP **Labiatæ**

(CATMINT, CATNEP)

Nepeta cataria

One of the best remedies for wind colic, especially in children and infants; produces gentle sleep. Also highly recommended for febrile; nervous, and infantile diseases, and to restore menstrual secretions. HHRM p. 66.

CEDRON SEED **Simarubaceæ**

Simaba cedron

An anti-spasmodic; used as a febrifuge in cases of intermittent fever.

CELANDINE **Papaveraceæ**

(GREATER CELANDINE)

Chelidonium majus

Used in scrofula, cutaneous diseases, piles, and affections of the spleen. Combined with Butternut Bark, as a purgative, it removes bile from the liver. It makes a most valuable anodyne ointment for sores. HHRM p. 67, *47.*

CELERY SEED **Umbelliferæ**

(SMALLAGE)

Apium graveolens

Much used in dropsical and liver troubles, and incontinence of urine; produces perspiration. HHRM p. 67.

CENTAURY **Gentianaceæ**

(EUROPEAN CENTAURY)

Erythræa centaurium, Centaurium erythræa

Expels worms. It is also very useful in autumnal fevers and dyspepsia, as well as to restore and regulate the menstrual flow.

CHAMOMILE FLOWERS, GERMAN **Compositæ**

(WILD CHAMOMILE, KAMILLE)

Matricaria chamomilla, Matricaria recutita

As a mild and gentle tonic and appetizer, the decoction is frequently served as a tea. It induces regular monthly periods, is excellent for the stomach and kidneys, and is useful in expelling worms. Externally it has been used with pronounced success as a wash for weak or irritated eyes. HHRM p. 68.

CHAMOMILE FLOWERS, ROMAN **Compositæ**

(COMMON CHAMOMILE, MANZANILLA, MAYTHEN)

Anthemis nobilis, Chamomilla nobilis, Chamæmelum nobile

Highly recommended for dyspepsia, weak stomach, hysteria, and nervousness; a most agreeable stomach tonic, increasing the desire for food. Relieves gas in the stomach, and favours perspiration and action of the kidneys. Useful in the treatment of colds and bronchitis. HHRM p. 68.

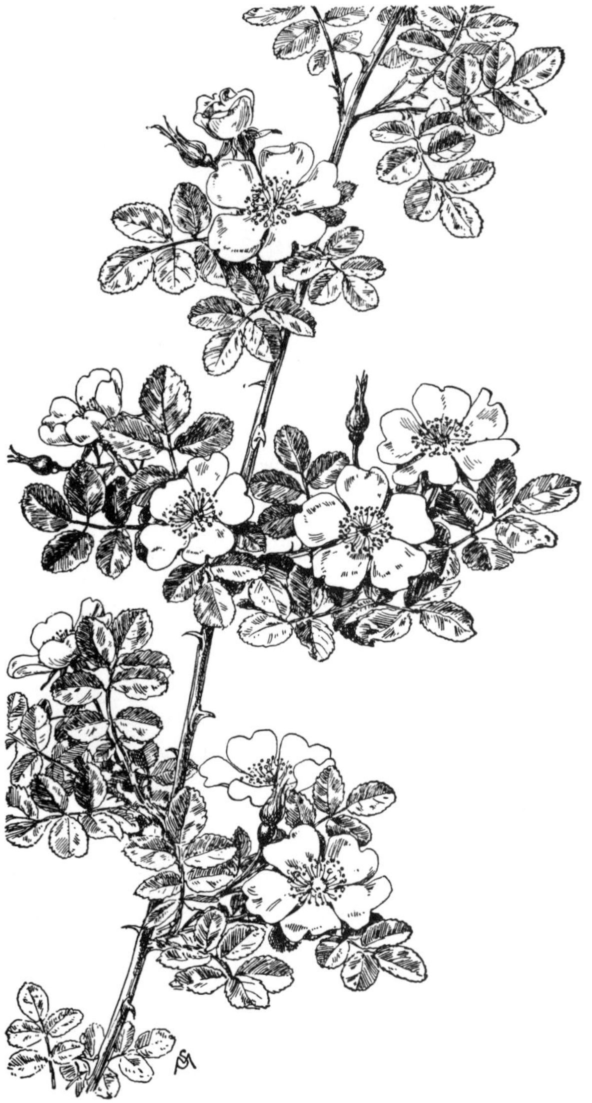

Sweetbrier, Brier Hips. Rosa rubiginosa.

4. **Brier Hips**, *page 27.*

CHERRY BARK, WILD **Rosaceæ**

Prunus virginiana, Prunus serotina

For coughs, bronchitis, asthma, etc.; valuable in all cases where it is desired to add tone and strength to the system, also in fever, diarrhea, jaundice, dyspepsia, scrofula, and general debility. HHRM p. 69.

CHESTNUT LEAVES **Cupuliferæ**

(SPANISH CHESTNUT)

Castanea vesca, Fagus castanea

An infusion of the leaves is highly recommended for whooping cough and may be taken freely. HHRM p. 60.

CHICKWEED **Caryophyllaceæ**

(STARWEED)

Stellaria media

An excellent blood purifier, very soothing to inflamed parts. Used as a poultice for old and indolent ulcers, also in ophthalmia, erysipelas, and cutaneous diseases. HHRM p. 69.

CHICORY ROOT **Compositæ**

(SUCCORY)

Cichorium intybus

Mildly tonic, laxative, and diuretic. Useful in disorders of the kidneys and liver, also for jaundice. Boiled with sugar to make Syrup of Succory, it is an excellent laxative for children, as it acts without irritation. HHRM p. 69.

CHIRETTA **Gentianaceæ**

(CHIRATA, INDIAN GENTIAN, INDIAN BALMONY)

Swertia chirata

Excellent in dyspepsia and as a tonic for general debility after fevers; cures constipation. Useful in liver affections as it promotes secretion of bile.

CHOCOLATE ROOT **Rosaceæ**

(NODDING AVENS, DROOPING AVENS, WATER AVENS, CURE ALL, WATER FLOWER, INDIAN CHOCOLATE, GEUM)

Geum rivale

One of the best astringent remedies for hemorrhage, dysentery, and chronic diarrhea, also useful for leucorrhea and other female complaints.

CLEAVERS **Rubiaceæ**

(CLIVERS, CATCHWEED, GOOSEGRASS)

Galium aparine

One of the most effective remedies for kidney and bladder troubles, and for suppression of urine; largely used in combination with Broom Tops, Uva-Ursi, and Buchu. The decoction is used as a wash to remove freckles.

CLOVER, RED **Leguminosæ (Fabaceæ)**

(TREFOIL, PURPLE CLOVER, SHAMROCK)

Trifolium pratense

Alterative and anti-spasmodic. A useful hot infusion in cases of bronchial and whooping cough. One of the best blood purifiers, especially favoured as a fomentation or poultice for local application where there is a tendency to cancerous growths and ulcers. *Illustration: p. 43.* HHRM p. 72.

CLOVER, WHITE **Leguminosæ (Fabaceæ)**

(TREFOIL, SWEET CLOVER, DUTCH CLOVER, SHAMROCK)

Trifolium repens

Useful for coughs and colds. Added to Mandrake, Senna, or Wormwood to give them a pleasant taste and prevent griping. Steeped in lard it makes an excellent salve for inflammations and burns. Celandine or Willow Bark may be added to this salve for their anodyne qualities. HHRM p. 73.

COLUMBO **Gentianaceæ**

(AMERICAN COLOMBO, AMERICAN CALUMBA)

Frasera carolinensis

Highly esteemed as a tonic and appetizer, giving tone and strength to the system. It is employed in rheumatism, dyspepsia, chronic diarrhea, cholera morbus, and cholera infantum, as well as in convalescence from fevers.

COLTSFOOT **Compositæ**

(COUGHWORT)

Tussilago farfara

Valuable in coughs, asthma, whooping cough, and pulmonary affections of every kind. Its demulcent qualities prove its efficacy in chronic coughs and consumption, being soothing and healing to the throat and lungs. It is also used in eases of scrofulous tumours, and is pulverized for administration as a snuff in cases of severe headache. HHRM p. 75.

COMFREY **Boraginaceæ**

Symphytum officinale

Esteemed as a remedy for catarrh, consumption, and pulmonary troubles, and also for diarrhea and dysentery, leucorrhea, and female debility, but better used to make salves and unguents for wounds. HHRM p. 75.

COOLWORT **Saxifragaceæ**

(MITREWORT, FOAM FLOWER)

Tiarella cordifolia, Mitella nuda

Very valuable in all bladder and kidney disorders, such as gravel, dropsy, and diabetes, and it is said to have no superior as a remedy for strangury.

CORIANDER SEED **Umbelliferæ**

(CILANTRO SEEDS, CHINESE PARSLEY SEEDS)

Coriandrum sativum

A warm cordial, giving tone to the stomach and strengthening the action of the heart. Has culinary uses. The leaves, called Cilantro or Chinese Parsley, are used fresh in cooking but lose much flavour when dried. HHRM p. 77.

CORN SILK **Graminaceæ**

(MAIZE)

Zea mays

A gentle diuretic and demulcent, acting mildly on the kidneys and bladder. Very beneficial in cystitis, catarrhal conditions of the urinary passages, gravel, or for painful urination from any cause.

CORSICA MOSS **Algæ**

(CORSICAN WORM MOSS)

Fucus helminthocorton, Alsidium helminthocorton

It is an excellent anthelmintic, and acts powerfully on intestinal worms.

COTTON ROOT **Malvaceæ**

Gossypium herbaceum

In diseases of the utero-genital organs it seems to evince its sole remedial virtues. It is a wonderful uterine tonic, invaluable in sterility, vaginitis, leucorrhea, menstrual irregularities and in cases of difficult parturition. As an abortifacient, its use is advised instead of ergot, since it promotes uterine contractions quite as efficiently, and without the bad after effects.

CRAMP BARK **Caprifoliaceæ**

(BLACK HAW, HOBBLE BUSH, DEVIL'S SHOE STRINGS, VIBURNUM, WITCHES' HOBBLE)

Viburnum alnifolium, Viburnum opulus, Viburnum prunifolium, Viburnum trilobum

One of the best remedies for female complaints. Very effective antispasmodic, relaxing to the cramps and pains incident to menstruation, pregnancy, and afterbirth. Used to treat spasms in asthma. HHRM p. 83.

CRAWL GRASS **Polygonaceæ**

(KNOT WEED, KNOT GRASS, LADIES THUMB)

Polygonum arenastrum, Polygonum persicaria

Astringent and vulnerary. Valued as a mouth wash and for the gums. Also said to be of benefit for diabetes, backache, and leg pains. HHRM p. 119.

CRAWLEY ROOT **Orchidaceæ**

(CHICKEN TOES, CORAL ROOT, DRAGON'S CLAW, FEVER ROOT, TURKEY CLAW)

Corallorhiza innata, Corallorhiza multiflora, Corallorhiza odontorhiza, Corallorhiza verna, Corallorhiza wistariana

Invaluable in suppression of lochia, typhoid, intermittent fevers, pleurisy, and night sweats; it breaks up colds and eases pain. HHRM p. 77, *71*.

CUBEB BERRIES **Piperaceæ**

(LOVE BERRIES, TAILED PEPPER)

Piper cubeba

Useful in bronchitis, coughs, and diseases of the urinary organs; gives tone to the stomach and is excellent in cases of wind colic. HHRM p. 80.

DAMIANA **Turneraceæ**

(LOVE HERB)

Turnera aphrodisiaca

Aphrodisiac, tonic, expectorant, stimulant, and laxative. HHRM p. 80.

DANDELION ROOT **Compositæ**

Taraxicum dens-leonis

A laxative that also increases the flow of urine. It is prescribed for jaundice and sluggish liver, also highly prized as a remedy for affections of the spleen and kidneys, dropsy, chronic costiveness, uterine obstructions, and as a purifier in diseases of the skin. HHRM p. 81.

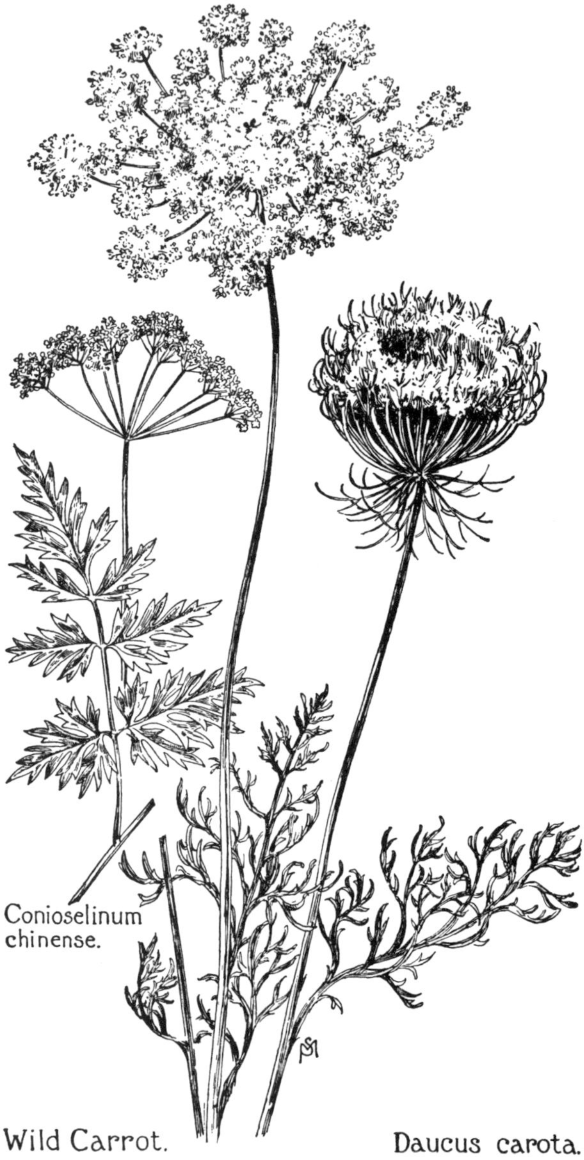

5. **Wild Carrot**, *page 31*.

DEER'S TONGUE **Compositæ**

(VANILLA LEAF)

Liatris odoratissima, Trilisa odorata, Trilisa odoratissima

Aromatic, tonic, demulcent, diaphoretic, and stimulant. HHRM p. 81.

DILL SEED **Umbelliferæ**

Anethum graveolens

A good stomachic, warm and grateful, expelling wind, and giving tone to the digestive system. Quiets the nerves, especially in babies with colic or gripes. The seeds are used with the leaves to flavour pickles. HHRM p. 85.

DOG GRASS **Gramineæ (Poaceæ)**

(COUCH GRASS, QUACK GRASS, QUITCH GRASS, TWITCH GRASS, WITCH GRASS)

Agropyron repens, Agropyrum repens, Elytrigia repens, Triticum repens

One of the best remedies for kidney and bladder troubles, often used with Cleavers, Uva-Ursi, and Buchu. HHRM p. 78.

DOGWOOD BARK **Cornaceæ**

(AMERICAN BOXWOOD, CORNEL, BUNCHBERRY, DWARF CORNEL)

Cornus florida, Cornus canadensis

An excellent substitute for Peruvian Bark, valuable in jaundice and liver complaints, and also useful in intermittent fevers. It is a mild tonic for the stomach, as well as a stimulant and an astringent. *Illustration: p. 48.*

ECHINACEA **Compositæ**

(BLACK SAMPSON, PURPLE CONEFLOWER, SAMPSON SNAKE ROOT)

Echinacea angustifolia, Echinacea pallida, Echinacea purpurea

Considered an excellent antiseptic alterative, it is a favourite ingredient of numerous blood purifiers. It increases the body's resistance to infection and septicæmia and it is used topically against boils, erysipelas, and piles. It is also an aphrodisiac and promotes perspiration. HHRM p. 175, *146.*

ELDER BERRIES **Caprifoliaceæ**

(POPGUN ELDER, COMMON ELDER)

Sambucus canadensis, Sambucus nigra, Sambucus racemosa

The berries are useful in rheumatism and are employed as a blood purifier in gouty affections. HHRM p. 89, *92.*

ELDER, DWARF **Caprifoliaceæ**

(DANEWORT, WALEWORT)

Sambucus ebulus

The leaves are valuable in gravel, dropsy, suppression of urine, and other kidney and bladder disorders. The root is a purgative. HHRM p. 89, *92*.

ELDER FLOWERS **Caprifoliaceæ**

(POPGUN ELDER, COMMON ELDER)

Sambucus canadensis, Sambucus nigra, Sambucus racemosa

As a hot tea, it increases the flow of urine, promotes expectoration, and causes sweating. It is also useful in erysipelas, constipation, and fevers. It is gently laxative and aperient. HHRM p. 89, *92*.

ELECAMPANE **Compositæ**

(ELF DOCK)

Inula helenium

Highly esteemed in dropsy, weakness of the digestive organs, and dyspepsia. As a powerful antiseptic and bactericide, it is also much used for coughs, colds, shortness of breath, lung troubles, and skin affections. HHRM p. 90.

ELM BARK, SLIPPERY **Ulmaceæ**

(MOOSE ELM, INDIAN ELM)

Ulmus fulva

Demulcent, emollient, expectorant, diuretic, and nutritive. Highly beneficial in dysentery diarrhea, inflammation of the throat, lungs, bowels, stomach, bladder, or kidneys; also effective when used as a poultice. HHRM p. 185.

EUCALYPTUS LEAVES **Myrtaceæ**

(BLUE GUM TREE, STRINGY BARK TREE)

Eucalyptus globulus

Antiseptic, disinfectant. Inhaled as vapour for lung troubles. HHRM p. 91.

EYEBRIGHT **Scrophulariaceæ**

(EUPHRASIA)

Euphrasia officinalis

Slightly tonic and astringent. Excellent for infusions or poultices in eye inflammations and catarrhal ophthalmia. Also good for hoarseness, coughs, earache, and headache that have supervened upon catarrhal affections.

FEMALE FERN **Athyriaceæ**

(LADY FERN)

Asplenium filix-femina, Athyrium filix-femina, Athyrium asplenioides

Used in expelling worms, especially tape worm. Similar in action to Male Fern, but gentler. HHRM p. 93.

FENNEL SEED **Umbelliferæ**

(FINOCCHIO, FINULE)

Fœniculum vulgare

Valued as a warming cordial; it expels the wind from the stomach. A galactagogue. Much used to flavour other herbal remedies. HHRM p. 93.

FENUGREEK **Leguminosæ (Fabaceæ)**

(FOENUGREEK)

Trigonella fœnum-græcum

A tea of the seed is useful as a gargle for sore throat and as a cooling drink in high fevers. The seeds boiled in milk will make thin people plump. As a poultice it is of benefit for wounds and inflammations. HHRM p. 93.

FEVERFEW **Compositæ**

(FEATHERFEW)

Chrysanthemum parthenium, Tanacetum parthenium, Matricaria parthenium

One of the oldest and best remedies for fevers, chills, and breaking up colds. The warm infusion is used also for headaches, flatulency, worms, irregular menstruation, hysterics, and suppression of the urine. HHRM p. 94, *71.*

FIGWORT **Scrophulariaceæ**

(THROATWORT, KNOTTED FIGWORT, WATER FIGWORT)

Scrophularia nodosa, Scrophularia aquatica

Has a diuretic affect on the kidneys. A fomentation or ointment is used for ulcers, piles, scrofula, cutaneous eruptions, abscesses, sores, and wounds.

FLAX SEED **Linaceæ**

(LINSEED)

Linum usitatissimum

An emollient, demulcent, pectoral alterative for colds, coughs, and irritation of the urinary organs. Excellent as a poultice for burns, boils, carbuncles, and old sores. Flax Seed oil is a mild, safe laxative. HHRM p. 96.

FLEABANE **Compositæ**

(BITTER WEED, CANADA FLEABANE, COLT'S TAIL, HORSE WEED)

Conyza canadensis, Erigeron canadense

Considered one of the most reliable remedies for dropsy, kidney troubles. Efficient also in diarrhea, diabetes, gravel, scalding urine, in hemorrhage of the bowels and uterus, and in bleeding wounds. HHRM p. 48.

FOXGLOVE **Scrophulariaceæ**

(DIGITALIS, FAIRY'S GLOVE, FAIRY THIMBLES)

Digitalis purpurea

An active remedy for too-rapid heart action; diuretic; valuable in Bright's disease; neuralgia, dropsy, acute inflammatory complaints, asthma, and febrile diseases. Care must be taken in its use as it is a poison.

FRINGE TREE **Oleaceæ**

(OLD MAN'S BEARD, CHIONATHUS, SNOWDROP TREE)

Chionanthus virginica

Aperient and diuretic, it has been used for years as a blood purifier and general tonic. It abates fever, acts as a gentle cathartic, is good for the kidneys, and makes an excellent alterative. An effective vulnerary, it may be applied as a poultice for inflammations or wounds.

FROSTWORT **Cistaceæ**

(CISTUS, FROSTWEED, ROCK ROSE)

Helianthemum canadense, Cistus canadensis

A superior alterative, and tonic remedy for all scrofulous diseases, syphilis, cancerous affections, and as a gargle in canker and scarlatina. It is used as an astringent wash in ophthalmia, itch, and cutaneous diseases. Excessive dosage may produce nausea or vomiting.

FUMITORY **Papaveraceæ (Fumariaceæ)**

(EARTH SMOKE, FUMUS)

Fumaria fungosa, Fumaria indica, Fumaria officinalis, Fumaria sempervirens

A mild tonic, weakly diaphoretic, useful as a diuretic and aperient. Acts on the bowels and kidneys, cleansing them from unhealthy secretions or obstructions; also useful in jaundice, scurvy, and in general debility of the digestive organs. When prepared as a tea, it is well to add powdered Anise or Fennel seed to it. HHRM p. 89, *71*.

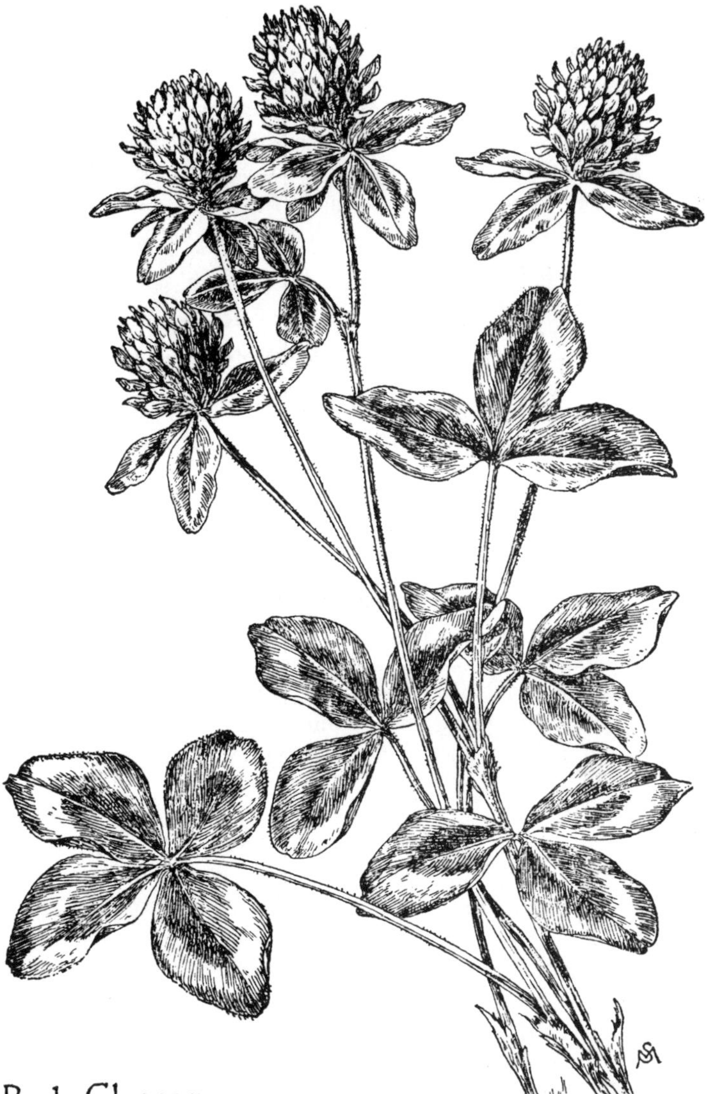

6. **Red Clover**, *page 35.*

GALANGAL **Zingiberaceæ**

(ALPINIA, CHEWING JOHN, COURT CASE ROOT, LITTLE JOHN TO CHEW, LOW JOHN ROOT, WILD GINGER)

Alpinia galangal, Alpinia officinarum

An aromatic stimulant. Taken as a tea it is carminative and reliably combats flatulence, dyspepsia, vomiting, and nervous stomach; it is also recommended as a remedy for sea-sickness. Powdered, it is used as a snuff for catarrh, nervous headache, and like complaints. HHRM p. 125.

GENTIAN **Gentianaceæ**

(BLUE GENTIAN, YELLOW GENTIAN, RATTLESNAKE ROOT, SAMPSON SNAKE ROOT)

Gentiana catesbæi, Gentiana lutea

One of the most powerful and valuable bitter tonics known; it improves the appetite, aids digestion, strengthens and tones up the entire system, and assists circulation. Very useful in dyspepsia, gout, scrofula, fever, and ague. It may be flavoured with Orange peel and Cardamom. HHRM p. 102.

GINGER, JAMAICA **Zingiberaceæ**

(JAMAICA GINGER, JAKE ROOT, WHITE GINGER, AFRICAN GINGER)

Zingiber officinale

Valuable in diarrhea, dysentery, flatulency, dyspepsia, water-brash, nervous stomach, migraine, vomiting, and to relieve pain in the bowels. A mild anodyne, it also prevents the griping of strong cathartics. HHRM p. 102.

GINSENG **Araliaceæ**

(FIVE FINGERS, SANG ROOT, WONDER OF THE WORLD)

Aralia quinquefolia, Panax quinquefolium

Demulcent and stomachic, useful in dyspepsia, loss of appetite, and nervous exhaustion. In China it is infused with drinks and taken with solid foods as a precautionary measure against sickness. HHRM p. 104, *92*.

GLOBE FLOWER **Ranunculaceæ**

(GLOBE RANUNCULUS, GLOBE TROLLIUS)

Trollius europæus

Tonic, febrifuge, aperient, anti-scorbutic, and diuretic. Used with success in intermittent and remittent fevers, it also forms an agreeable bitters employed in coughs and gravel. Combines well with White Clover.

GOATS RUE **Leguminosæ (Fabaceæ)**

(DEVIL'S THONGS, CAT'S GUT)

Galega officinalis, Cracca virginiana, Tephrosia virginiana, Tephrosium virginiana

A gentle diaphoretic stimulant. Excellent in case of fevers, it provokes sweating and tends to overcome the effect of disease if taken inwardly; also expels worms. Continued use of the decoction is said to be very effective in enlarging the bust, acting as a glandular tonic. HHRM p. 83.

GOBERNADORA **Zygophyllaceæ**

(CHAPARRAL, CREOSOTE BUSH)

Larrea tridentata

Anti-bacterial, anti-fungal, anti-inflammatory, disinfectant, and vulnerary. Employed for baths and fomentations in rheumatism. Also used for gastric disturbances and gallstones. Because of its remarkable antiseptic properties, it is often applied as a fomentation to pains, aches, sprains, bruises, sores, cuts, and wounds. It can be made into a salve, too.

GOLDEN ROD **Compositæ**

(WOUNDWORT, AARON'S ROD)

Solidago virgaurea

Aromatic, stimulant, carminative, and vulnerary. A good diaphoretic when taken in the form of a warm infusion, useful in cases where sweating is desired, as in breaking up colds and fevers. Also helpful in dysmenorrhea and amenorrhea. *Illustration: p. 53.*

GOLDEN SEAL **Ranunculaceæ**

(YELLOW PUCCOON)

Hydrastis canadensis

A highly esteemed remedy for catarrh, also female complaints. It is a powerful tonic at the same time, exerting an especial influence upon the mucous surfaces and tissues. HHRM p. 104.

GOLD THREAD **Ranunculaceæ**

(MOUTHROOT)

Coptis trifolia

An old and reliable remedy for canker in the mouth and stomach. Valuable as a gargle in ulcerations of the throat. Used as a local application in thrush or yeast infection of the mouth, for children.

GRAINS OF PARADISE **Zingibigeraceæ**

(GUINEA GRAINS, MELAGUETA PEPPER)

Aframomum melegueta, Amomum granum-paradisi, Ampelopsis melegueta

A warming stimulant, digestive aid, and diuretic. HHRM p. 107.

GRAVEL ROOT **Compositæ**

(AGUE WEED, JOE-PYE WEED, QUEEN OF THE MEADOW)

Eupatorium purpureum

Much used for kidney and bladder troubles, and in combination with Uva-Ursi it is a superior remedy in lithic gravel. HHRM p. 108, *92*.

GROUND IVY **Labiatæ**

(ALEHOOF, GILL-GO-OVER-THE-GROUND)

Glechoma hederacea

Stimulant, tonic, and pectoral; useful in asthma, diseases of the lungs and kidneys, and jaundice. The sweetened infusion, called Gill Tea, is anti-scorbutic, relieves headache and coughs, and is pleasingly aromatic.

GUAIAC WOOD **Zygophyllaceæ**

(LIGNUM VITÆ)

Guaiacum officinale

Mild laxative and diuretic, useful in rheumatism, rheumatoid arthritis, gout, and painful or suppressed menstruation. The powder is given for tonsillitis.

GUARANA **Sapindaceæ**

(PAULLINIA)

Paullinia cupana

Stimulant, aphrodisiac, tonic, excitant, and nervine. Used in headaches.

GUM PLANT **Compositæ**

(SCALY GRINDELIA, ROSIN WEED, GRINDELIA ROBUSTA)

Grindelia camporum, Grindelia cuneifolia, Grindelia squarrosa

Good for asthma, bronchitis, whooping cough, and catarrh of the bladder. Large doses irritate the kidneys. Apply externally to burns and blisters.

HAIRCAP MOSS **Polytrichaceæ**

(BEAR'S BED, ROBIN'S EYE, GROUND MOSS)

Polytrichium juniperum, Polytrichum commune

A vigorous diuretic for dropsy, gravel, and all kidney and urinary troubles.

HAWTHORN **Rosaceæ**

Cratægus oxycantha

Supportive to those with a weak heart or poor circulation. HHRM p. 110.

HEAL ALL **Labiatæ**

(SELF- HEAL, ALL HEAL, WOUNDWORT)

Prunella vulgaris

An astringent, valuable in cases of hemorrhage and also as a gargle or mouth wash in cases of canker and sore throat. HHRM p. 180, *146*.

HELONIAS **Liliaceæ**

(FALSE UNICORN ROOT, STARWORT)

Chamælirium luteum, Helonias lutea

Tonic, diuretic; in large doses emetic. Valuable in leucorrhea, amenorrhea, and dysmenorrhea, and to remove the tendency to repeated and successive miscarriage. Useful in male impotence; a urogenital tonic. HHRM p. 200.

HEMLOCK **Umbelliferæ**

(BEAVER POISON, POISON HEMLOCK, POISON PARSLEY)

Conium maculatum

Sedative, anti-spasmodic, narcotic poison that brings on complete paralysis, loss of speech, asphyxia, and death; anodyne poultice in cancerous ulcers.

HENNA **Lythraceæ**

(AL-KHANNA, MEHNDI)

Lawsonia alba, Lawsonia inermis

Used as a dye for the hair. Applied topically for affections of the skin.

HICKORY BARK **Juglandaceæ**

(SHAGBARK HICKORY)

Carya ovata

A gentle cathartic, also used as a wash for ulcers and sore eyes. The boiled bark applied warm as a cloth-wrapped fomentation brings arthritis relief.

HOPS **Urticaceæ**

Humulus lupulus

A valuable sedative; produces quiet sleep, even in cases of nervousness. As a poultice, gives relief from local pains, such as swellings. HHRM p. 113.

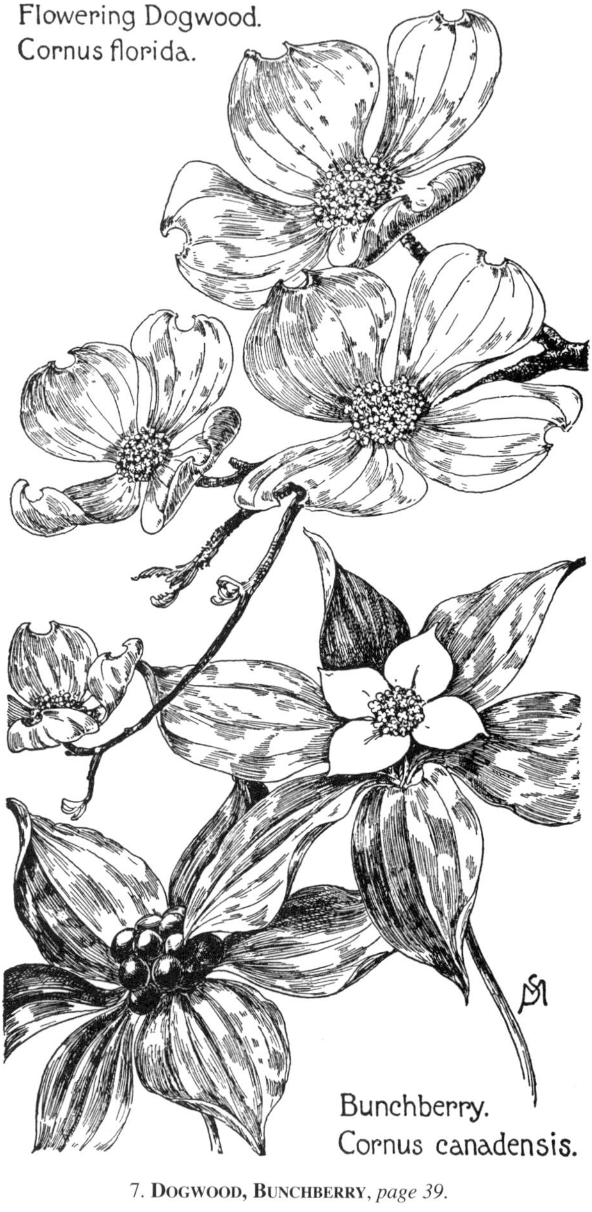

7. **Dogwood, Bunchberry**, *page 39.*

HOREHOUND **Labiatæ**

(WHITE HOREHOUND, HOARHOUND)

Marrubium vulgare

An old and highly valued expectorant and tonic remedy for coughs, asthma, laryngitis, bronchitis, and all pulmonary troubles; the cold infusion is also used in dyspepsia and water-brash, and as a vermifuge. HHRM p. 114.

HORSEMINT **Labiatæ**

(MONARDA LUTEA, SPOTTED MONARDA)

Mentha sylvestris, Monarda punctata

Aromatic, pungent, and bitter. Also useful as a carminative, stimulant, emmenagogue, nervine, diaphoretic, and diuretic; indicated in cases of nausea, colic, rheumatism, neuralgia, and diarrhea. HHRM p. 134, *122*.

HORSENETTLE ROOT **Solanaceæ**

(BULL NETTLE, TREADFOOT, SAND BRIER, APPLE OF SODOM, POISONOUS POTATO)

Solanum carolinense

Anodyne, diuretic, and aphrodisiac. It is useful in treating epilepsy and blood impurities as well as in kidney and bladder affections.

HORSERADISH **Cruciferæ**

(MOUNTAIN RADISH, GREAT RAIFORT, RED COLE)

Cochlearia armoracia

Much used as a remedy for colic and bladder troubles; also in cases of rheumatism, paralysis, dropsy, and scurvy.

HORSETAIL GRASS **Equisetaceæ**

(SHAVE-GRASS, BOTTLE-BRUSH, DUTCH RUSHES)

Equisetum arvense, Equisetum hyemale, Equisetum sylvaticum

Diuretic, astringent; prized for dropsy, gleet, gravel, kidney, and bladder troubles. Also an emmenagogue and an effective wash for putrid wounds.

HOUND'S TONGUE **Boraginaceæ**

(DOG'S TONGUE)

Cynoglossum officinal, Lindefolia spectabilis

Valuable for coughs, catarrh, bleeding from the lungs, and disorganizations of the respiratory apparatus. As a sitting-bath, the infusion is good for piles.

HYDRANGEA **Saxifragaceæ**

(WILD HYDRANGEA, SEVEN BARKS, COMMON HYDRANGEA)

Hydrangea arborescens

Highly recommended for kidney trouble and to remove gravel and mineral deposits from the bladder, relieving the excruciating pains caused thereby.

HYSSOP **Labiatæ**

Hyssopus officinalis

A gentle expectorant, diaphoretic, and stimulant tonic; quieting to pain; valuable in quinsy, catarrh, asthma, and chest diseases. HHRM p. 114.

ICELAND MOSS **Parmeliaceæ**

(CETRARIA, ICELAND LICHEN)

Cetraria islandica

Used in chronic catarrh, dysentery, and diarrhea and as a gentle tonic in dyspepsia and during convalescence from exhausting diseases.

INDIAN HEMP, BLACK **Apocynaceæ**

(CANADIAN HEMP, HEMP DOGBANE, PRAIRIE DOGBANE)

Apocynum cannabinum

Diuretic, diaphoretic, expectorant; quiets and eases pain; used in dropsy resulting from heart failure, intermittent and remittent fevers, pneumonia, and obstructions of the kidneys. An overdose will lead to vomiting.

INDIAN PHYSIC **Rosaceæ**

(BOWMAN'S ROOT, AMERICAN IPECACUANHA, GILLENIA)

Gillenia trifoliata, Spiræa trifoliata, Spireæa stipulata

A tonic and gentle physic, much used in croup; also considered valuable in rheumatism, dropsy, dyspepsia, chronic costiveness, and for relieving suppression of the menses. In higher doses it is an emetic and a vermifuge.

INDIAN TURNIP **Araceæ**

(JACK-IN-THE-PULPIT, WILD TURNIP, PEPPER TURNIP, DRAGON ROOT, DEVIL'S EAR, MEMORY ROOT)

Arum triphyllum, Arisame triphyllum

Much used as a physic in liver troubles; also highly recommended in croup, cough, asthma, bronchitis, pain in the chest and similar affections; also for colic, low typhoid and externally in scrofulous troubles, and scald-head.

INDIGO, WILD **Leguminosæ**

(BAPTISIA, HORSE-FLY WEED, RATTLEBUSH, INDIGO-WEED)

Baptisia tinctoria, Sophora tinctoria, Podalyria tinctoria

Internally purgative, emetic, and astringent, it makes a valuable antiseptic wash or gargle for all species of skin ulcers, sore mouth, putrescent throat, fetid leucorrhea, urethral discharge, and for old sores which refuse to heal.

IRISH MOSS **Algæ**

(CARRAGEEN, IRISH SEA MOSS, PEARL MOSS)

Chondrus crispus

A demulcent used in coughs, colds, pulmonary affections, diarrhea, dysentery, and rickets. Boiled in milk it is a nutritive tonic. HHRM p. 115.

IRONWEED ROOT **Compositæ**

(VERNONIA, PRAIRIE IRONWEED)

Vernonia fasciculata, Vernonia noveboracensis, Vernonia gigantea

A bitter tonic, aperient, deobstruent, and alterative, useful for diabetes, aids in the reduction of persistent fever and chronic headache; regulates the menstrual cycle and acts as a blood purifier. *Illustration: p. 58.*

JABORANDI **Rutaceæ**

(ARRUDA BRAVA, JAMGUARANDI, JUARANDI)

Pilocarpus jaborandi

Causes profuse sweating. Excellent for breaking up colds, good for rheumatism, Bright's disease, and influenza. As a constituent of tonics to be applied to the hair and scalp, it is much valued since it stimulates the growth of the hair and gives health to the scalp.

JALAP **Convolvulaceæ**

(BINDWEED, HIGH JOHN, JOHN THE CONQUEROR, KING OF THE WOODS, KING ROOT, MAN OF THE EARTH, MAN ROOT)

Ipomœa jalapa, Ipomœa pandurata, Ipomœa purga, Convolvulus jalapa, Convolvulus panduratus

An irritant and cathartic hydragogue, operating energetically and producing liquid stools. It is best employed in long-standing cases of intestinal torpor and when combined with carminatives like Ginger. It may also be combined with Wormwood or Wormseed for use as a vermifuge. In intestinal inflammations it should not be used. HHRM p. 111.

JESSAMINE, YELLOW **Loganiaceæ**

(YELLOW JASMINE, FALSE JASMINE, WILD WOODBINE, CAROLINA JESSAMINE)

Gelsemium nitidum, Gelsemium sempervirens

A valuable febrifuge in all except congestive fevers; also useful in nervous irritability, headache, tetanus, and to promote contractions of the uterus, but its use is greatly restricted because in high doses it is a fatal poison.

JEZEBEL ROOT **Iridaceæ**

(ORRIS ROOT, LOUISIANA IRIS, SWEET IRIS)

Iris foliosa, Iris fulva, Iris hexagona, Iris tectorum, etc.

Excellent remedy for cystitis, bladder troubles, calculous affections such as gravel, and chronic inflammation of the kidneys; it is also used for leucorrhea, dropsy, and rheumatism. HHRM p. 116.

JOB'S TEARS **Gramineæ (Poaceæ)**

(TEAR GRASS, BEAD PLANT)

Coix lacryma-jobi

Mainly strung as beads which, worn by children at the teething period, relieve and obviate much danger and distress at that time. Also offered in case of goiter, to be worn persistently. HHRM p. 117.

JUNIPER BERRIES **Coniferæ**

(GINEPRO)

Juniperus communis

Used for years as a remedy for kidney and bladder troubles in combination with Broom Tops, Uva-Ursi, and Cleavers. Efficacious in gonorrhea, gleet, leucorrhea, dropsy, and kidney complaints in general. HHRM p. 118.

KAVA KAVA **Piperaceæ**

(AVA, INTOXICATING PEPPER, AVA PEPPER)

Piper methysticum

Calming, relaxing, mild anodyne; a remedy for gout and venereal diseases.

KIDNEYWORT **Crassulaceæ**

(WALL PENNYWORT, PENNY PIES)

Cotyledon umbilicus

Acts with marked benefit on the kidneys, used also with excellent results for asthma and epilepsy.

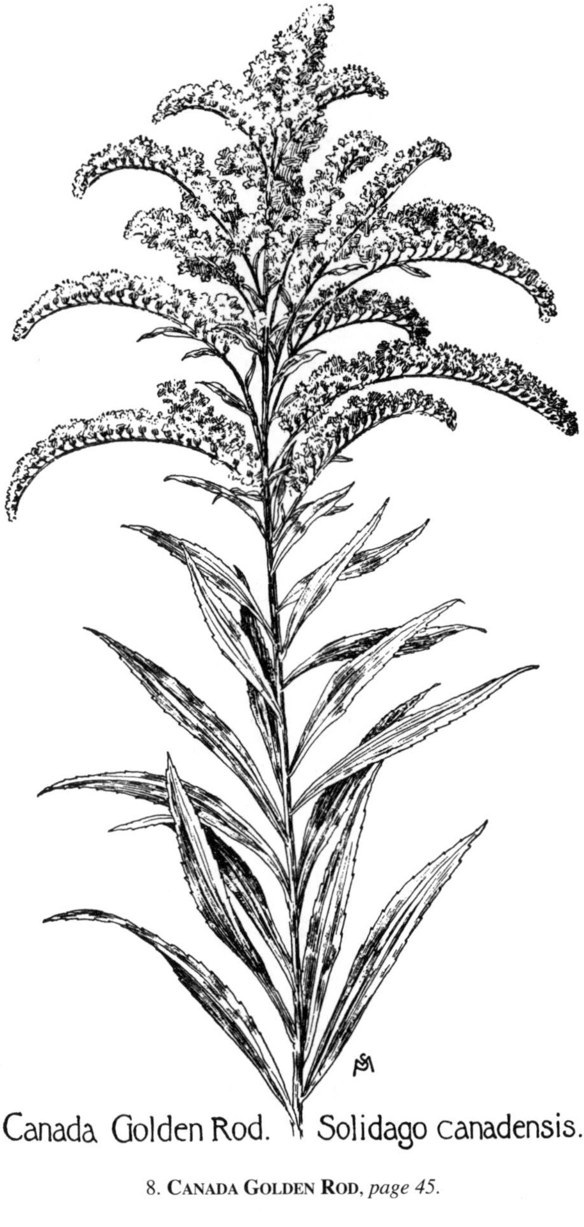

8. **Canada Golden Rod**, *page 45.*

KNOTGRASS **Polygonaceæ**

(CENTINODE, NINETY-KNOT, NINE-JOINTS)

Polygonum aviculare

Efficacious in expelling gravel from the kidneys and bladder; eases strangury. Dissolves phlegm. Astringent wash for piles. HHRM p. 119.

KOLA NUTS **Sterculiaceæ**

(KOLA SEEDS, GURRU NUTS, BISSY NUTS, COLA SEEDS)

Cola acuminata, Kola vera, Sterculia acuminata

Stimulant, tonic, nervine, diuretic, astringent; contains caffeine; not unlike Coca in its ability to aid endurance of fatigue without food; useful in neuralgia, headache, migraine, indigestion, weak and irregular heartbeat.

KOUSSO **Rosaceæ**

(KOOSO)

Hagenia Abyssinica, Banksia abyssinica, Brayera anthelmintica

Anthelmintic. In the proper dosage, if taken with Lemon-juice water after a 24-48 hour fast, it is a specific for expelling tapeworms. An overdose may produce nausea and vomiting as a side effect.

LABRADOR TEA **Ericaceæ**

(SAINT JAMES'S TEA)

Ledum latifolium, Ledum groenlandicum

Recommended for coughs and as a tonic, increasing the desire for food; also useful in dyspepsia, dysentery, and skin diseases.

LADY'S BEDSTRAW **Rubiaceæ**

(CHEESE RENNING, YELLOW BEDSTRAW)

Galium verum

Highly prized for its soothing and healing qualities to inflamed surfaces including irritated throat, bowels, kidneys, and urinary organs. The fresh juice makes a poultice for boils. Used to curdle cheese and colour it yellow.

LADY'S MANTLE **Rosaceæ**

(LION'S FOOT, NINE HOOKS, LEONTOPODIUM, STELLARIA)

Alchemilla vulgaris

Astringent, styptic, vulnerary; stops bleeding and vomiting. Halts excessive menstruation if taken as both tea and douche. Do not use while pregnant.

LAMB'S QUARTERS **Chenopodiaceæ**

(WHITE GOOSEFOOT, MUTTON TOPS, DIRTWEED, PIGWEED, BACONWEED, FAT HEN)

Chenopodium album

Anthelmintic, anti-spasmodic, and carminative when used in combination with other herbs. Fresh, it is an excellent pot-herb when served with butter.

LARKSPUR **Ranunculacæ**

(LARK'S HEEL, LARK'S CLAW, KNIGHT'S SPUR, DELPHINIUM)

Delphinium consolida

Ointment made from leaves and ground seeds applied externally to destroy insects on the body such as lice and scabies. Do not ingest; it is a poison.

LAVENDER **Labiatæ**

Lavandula officinalis

Valuable in flatulency, fainting, and to arrest vomiting; usually combined with other medicines. Much liked for its fragrance; used to scent cosmetics. In sachets, it keeps moths from clothing, linens, and furs. HHRM p. 120.

LETTUCE, WILD **Compositæ**

(LACTUCARIUM, LETTUCE OPIUM)

Lactuca virosa

Highly esteemed to quiet coughing and allay nervous irritation. As an anodyne, soporific sedative it is a good, safe remedy to produce sleep.

LICORICE ROOT **Leguminosæ**

Glycyrrhiza glabra, Glycyrrhiza glanuldifera, Glycyrrhiza echinata

Excellent for coughs, asthma, and bronchial affections, as well as irritation of the urinary organs and pain of the intestines in diarrhea. HHRM p. 124.

LIFE EVERLASTING **Compositæ**

(PEARLY EVERLASTING)

Gnaphalium spp., Antenneria spp., Anaphalis spp.

Anodyne, astringent, and pectoral; a favourite remedy for diarrhea, as well as coughs, colds, and catarrh of the lungs, and to produce perspiration. Ulcerations of the mouth and throat should be relieved by chewing the fresh tops and swallowing the juice. The dried herb combines well with Hops as a poultice for sprains, bruises, boils, painful swellings. HHRM p. 125, 2.

LIFE ROOT **Compositæ**

(GOLDEN GROUNDSEL, SQUAW WEED, GOLDEN SENECIO)

Senecio aureus

Valuable for strangury, gravel, and kidney complaints; a very efficient emmenagogue in cases of female irregularities, and noted for the peculiar influence it has upon the female reproductive organs. Useful as a pectoral.

LILY OF THE VALLEY ROOT **Liliaceæ**

(MAY LILY, CONVALLARIA, OUR LADY'S TEARS, LADDER-TO-HEAVEN, JACOB'S LADDER, MALE LILY)

Convallaria magalis

In small doses it strengthens the heart, quickly relieving the shortness of breath and palpitations of heart disease, and after having given it for 2 or 3 days, it may be stopped for a week or more without the symptoms returning. It increases the flow of urine and reduces dropsy.

LILY ROOT **Liliaceæ**

(MADONNA LILY)

Lilium candidum

Employed with good results for dropsy and kidney troubles; also useful in dysentery, diarrhea, and leucorrhea. Combined with Wild Cherry Bark it is used for bronchial affections. Used externally as a poultice for boils, skin eruptions, and scrofulous ulcers.

LINDEN FLOWERS **Tiliaceæ**

LINN FLOWERS, LIME TREE, TILLEUL)

Tilia europoea, Tilia vulgaris, Tilia intermedia, Tilia cordata, Tilia platyphylla

Acts favourably on the kidneys and bladder, and in female complaints. As a tea it soothes indigestion, and when in combination with Mint and Horehound, it relieves laryngitis. The infusion prepared as a warm bath settles hysteria. The fomentation is a good poultice for painful swellings.

LIVERWORT **Peltigeraceæ**

(ASH-COLOURED GROUND LIVERWORT)

Peltigera canina, Lichen caninus, Lichen cinereus terrestris

One of the old reliable diuretic home remedies for disorders of kidneys, also used for dropsy, fevers, hepatic complaints, bleeding of the lungs, and coughs. May also be employed as a vulnerary poultice.

LOBELIA **Lobeliaceæ**

(RAPUNTIUM INFLATUM, INDIAN-TOBACCO, PUKEWEED, ASTHMA WEED, GAGROOT, VOMITWORT, BLADDERPOD, EYEBRIGHT)

Lobelia inflata

A household remedy, unexcelled for breaking up colds, bronchial affections, and croup. Invaluable in spasmodic asthma, pneumonia, catarrh, cramps, hysteria, and convulsions. Used externally as a poultice for sprains, bruises, felons, and the stings of insects.

LOGWOOD CHIPS **Leguminosæ**

(BLOODWOOD, PEACHWOOD)

Hæmatoxylon campeachianum, Hæmatoxylon lignum

A strong astringent and an excellent tonic used with good effect in cases of chronic diarrhea, and other cases where such a remedy is needed. It is largely used in dyeing.

LOVAGE **Umbelliferæ**

(BO' HOG ROOT, GOUT WEED, LAVOSE, SMELLAGE)

Levisticum officinale, Ligusticum levisticum, Ligusticum actæifolium, Ligusticum cornubiense, Ligusticum podograria

Aromatic, stimulant, diuretic, carminative, deobstruent, and sudorific. Combined with other medicines as a corrective for flavour. Used in female complaints to relieve suppressed menstruation. HHRM p. 129.

LUNGWORT **Lobariaceæ**

(TREE LUNGWORT, OAK LUNGS, LUNG LICHEN, LUNG MOSS)

Lobaria pulmonaria, Sticta pulmonaria

One of the most valuable remedies for lung troubles, asthma, colds, coughs, influenza, bronchitis, and nasal catarrh. It makes a good vulnerary poultice.

LYCOPODIUM **Lycopodiaceæ**

(CLUB MOSS, VEGETABLE SULPHUR, WOLF'S CLAW)

Lycopodium clavatum, Muscus clavatum, Muscus terrestris repens

Diuretic and anti-spasmodic; it is useful in rheumatism, epilepsy, dysentery, and renal disorders. The powdered spores may be dusted on the skin in various cutaneous diseases such as eczema and erysipelas. Also dusted on excoriated, scraped, or chapped skin and to prevent chafing in infants.

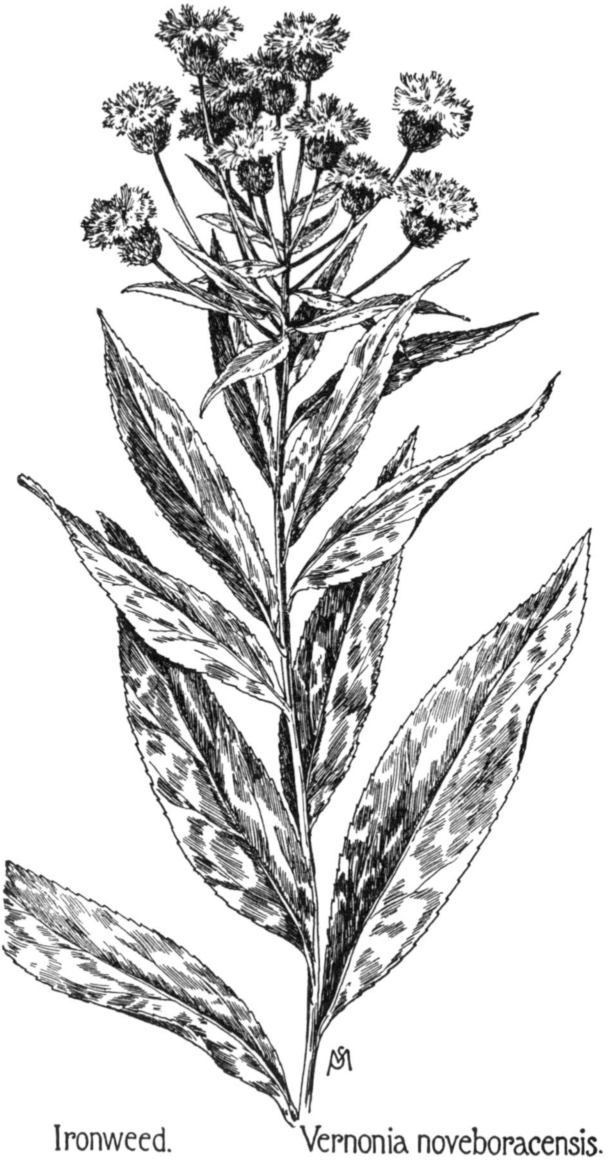

9. **Ironweed**, *page 51*.

MACE **Myristicaceæ**

(MACIS, MUSCADIER)

Myristica fragrans, Myristica moschata, Myristica officinalis

Aromatic flavouring agent; helps digestion. If taken to excess it may bring on over-excitement. HHRM p. 130.

MAGNOLIA BARK **Magnoliaceæ**

Magnolia glauca, Magnolia grandiflora, Magnolia macrophylla

An excellent bitter tonic, warm and aromatic; it is also anti-periodic and valuable in intermittent fevers, dyspepsia, dysentery, erysipelas, leucorrhea, and as a wash for tetter and salt rheum. HHRM p. 131.

MA HUANG **Ephedraceæ**

(EPHEDRA, NEVADA JOINT-FIR, DESERT TEA, MORMON TEA)

Ephedra intermedia, Ephedra sinensis, Ephedra distacha, Ephedra nevadensis

Alterative, diuretic, stimulant, decongestant, bronchial dilator, and appetite suppressor, it is of benefit in asthma, bronchitis, hay fever, and nasal cattarh.

MAIDENHAIR FERN **Aspleniaceæ**

(HAIR OF VENUS)

Asplenium trichomanes, Adiantum capillus-veneris, Adiantum raddianum

A most highly valued remedy for chronic catarrh of the lungs, bronchitis, croup, coughs, asthma, hoarseness, influenza, pleurisy, jaundice, febrile diseases, and erysipelas. HHRM p. 93.

MALE FERN **Dryopteridaceæ**

(MALE SHIELD FERN)

Dryopteris felix-mas, Aspidium filix-mas

A valuable anthelmintic, used to expel tapeworm. HHRM p. 93.

MANDRAKE ROOT, AMERICAN **Berberidaceæ**

(MAY APPLE, WILD LEMON, RACCOONBERRY, HOG APPLE)

Podophyllum peltatum

One of the best regulators for liver and bowels; a sure physic, often mixed with Senna leaves, valuable in jaundice, bilious and intermittent fever, or wherever a powerful cathartic is required. Small doses only should be given, in large doses it can produce nausea, vomiting, inflammation of the stomach and intestines, and fatal collapse. HHRM p. 132, *122*.

MANNA ASH **Oleaceæ**

(FLAKE MANNA)

Fraxinus ornus

Demulcent, nutritive, and laxative; suitable for costive children.

MAPLE, RED **Aceraceæ**

(SWAMP MAPLE, CURLED MAPLE)

Acer rubrum

Gentle tonic also used as a mild astringent wash for sore eyes.

MARIGOLD, CALENDULA **Compositæ**

(POT MARIGOLD)

Calendula officinalis, Caltha officinalis

One of the valuable remedies in fever, scrofula, jaundice and female complaints. Used internally and externally for wounds. HHRM p. 63.

MARJORAM, SWEET **Labiatæ**

(KNOTTED MARJORAM)

Origanum marjorana

Acts as a tonic, very effective in combination with Chamomile or Gentian. Promotes perspiration and menstruation, and relieves eruptive diseases. Also employed as a culinary flavouring agent. HHRM p. 132.

MARSHMALLOW ROOT **Malvaceæ**

(HOLLYHOCK, MALLOW, ALTHÆA ROOT, ROSE OF SHARON)

Althæa officinalis, Althæa rosea, Althæa rosa-sinensis, Althæa zebrina, etc., also *Malva alcea* and many other *Malva spp.*

Soothing and healing to inflamed bowels, valuable in hoarseness, catarrh, pneumonia, strangury, gravel, and all kidney complaints, and as a poultice for painful swellings, including felon and herpetic whitlow. See also Althæa Leaf. HHRM p. 28.

MASTERWORT **Umbelliferæ**

(IMPERIAL MASTERWORT, RULER'S ROOT)

Imperatoria ostruthium, Peucedanum ostruthium

Sialagogue, stimulant, anti-spasmodic, carminative, and stomachic; of use in flatulency, dyspepsia, asthma, painful or suppressed menstruation, and other menstrual complaints. HHRM p. 133.

MATÉ **Aquifoliaceæ**

(YERBA MATE, CHIMARRÃO, CIMARRÓN)

Ilex paraguariensis

Tonic and stimulant. A real health tea, and the finest substitute for ordinary tea or coffee. An astringent cerebral excitant imported from South America, it is well worth sampling as an agreeable beverage. Also used externally as a wash for sores and ulcers.

MATICO **Piperaceæ**

(SOLDIER'S HERB)

Piper angustifolium, Piper granulosum, Piper elongatum

An aromatic stimulant. Useful to arrest discharges from mucous surfaces, such as leucorrhoea, gonorrhea, and bacterial catarrh of the bladder.

MEADOWSWEET **Rosaceæ**

(HARDHACK, QUEEN OF THE MEADOW)

Spiræa tomentosa, Spiræa ulmaria, Filipendula ulmaria, Filipendula vulgaris

Anodyne and diuretic. A reliable remedy in dropsy, strangury, gravel, urinary disorders, diarrhea, dysentery, and debility of the bowels. Improves digestion. Aids lame back and neuralgia. *Illustration: p. 63.* HHRM p. 160.

MEZEREON **Thymelæaceæ**

(FLOWERING SPURGE, PARADISE PLANT)

Daphne mezereum

Cathartic, deobstruent, stimulant, and vesicant.

MILKWEED **Asclepiadaceæ**

(BUTTERFLY BUSH, SWAMP MILKWEED, PLEURISY ROOT)

Asclepias incarnata, Asclepias syriaca

Anodyne; it produces expectoration and relieves cough and pain in asthma and pleurisy. Used in amenorrhea and other female complaints. Acts freely on the bowels and kidneys, hence recommended for dropsy and retention of urine. Also valued for use in scrofulous troubles. HHRM p. 61, *71*.

MISTLETOE **Loranthaceæ**

Viscum album

Nervine narcotic; used to treat spasmodic nervous complaints, also to stop bloody flux. Too great a dose may bring on convulsions. HHRM p. 135.

MOUSE EAR **Compositæ**

(HAWKWEED, PILOSELLA)

Hieracium pilosella

Prized as a remedy for kidney and bladder troubles, also useful in coughs, diarrhea, and bowel obstructions.

MUGWORT **Compositæ**

Artemisia vulgaris

Useful in female complaints in combination with Marigold Flowers, Cramp Bark, and Black Haw; recommended for epilepsy and hysteria, and to promote perspiration and increase the flow of urine. HHRM p. 136.

MUIRA PUAMA **Olacaceæ**

(MARAPUAMA, POTENCY WOOD)

Ptychopetalum olacoides, Ptychopetalum uncinatum

Nervine, stimulant, and aphrodisiac; a male tonic.

MULLEIN FLOWERS **Scrophulariaceæ**

(BLANKET HERB, TORCHES)

Verbascum thapsis

Quiets pain, produces sleep; in larger doses, a laxative. HHRM p. 136, *122*.

MULLEIN LEAVES **Scrophulariaceæ**

(BLANKET HERB, TORCHES)

Verbascum thapsis

Esteemed in asthma, croup, and bronchitis. Valuable in dysentery and piles. A poultice in swollen joints, mumps, and sore throat. HHRM p. 136, *122*.

MUSTARD SEED **Cruciferæ**

(BLACK MUSTARD, BROWN MUSTARD, RED MUSTARD, YELLOW MUSTARD, WHITE MUSTARD)

Brassica juncea, Brassica nigra, Sinapis juncea, Sinapis nigra
Brassica alba, Brassica hirta, Sinapis alba, Sinapis hirta

The whole seed is used as a tonic in dyspepsia. HHRM p. 137.

MYRRH, GUM **Burseraceæ**

Commiphora molmol, Commiphora myrrha

Astringent, expectorant, and vulnerary. HHRM p. 138.

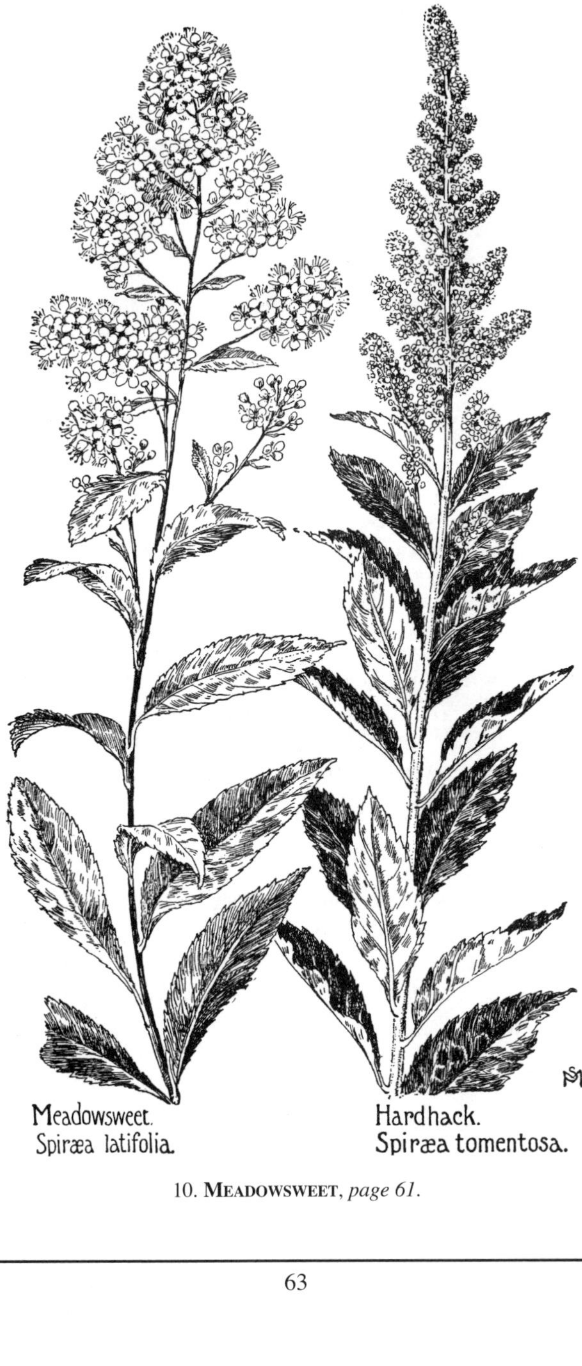

10. MEADOWSWEET, *page 61*.

NERVE ROOT **Orchidaceæ**

(LADY'S SLIPPER, NOAH'S ARK, YELLOW LADY'S SLIPPER)

Cypripedium pubescens, Cyprepedium parviflorum

A very gentle stimulant and tonic, invaluable in nervousness, headaches, hysterics, and all cases of nervous irritability. Excellent also for neuralgia and rheumatism. HHRM p. 120, *92.*

NETTLE LEAVES **Urticaceæ**

(STINGING NETTLE)

Urtica dioica

Valuable in diarrhea, dysentery, hemorrhoids, hemorrhages, and scrobutic affections, or in overcoming a tendency to scurvy. HHRM p. 139.

OLIBANUM, GUM **Burseraceæ**

(FRANKINCENSE)

Boswellia carteri, Boswellia thurifera

Known as an incense, it is also a stimulant. Inhaling steam from water in which the resin is boiled relieves bronchitis and laryngitis. Chewing a grain or two of the resin sweetens the breath. HHRM p. 97.

ORRIS ROOT **Iridaceæ**

(IRIS ROOT, LOVE ROOT, QUEEN ELIZABETH ROOT)

Iris florentina, Iris germanica

Effective for coughs, laryngitis, hoarseness, and affections of the lungs, but more prized for its fragrance, which resembles violets. Used to sweeten offensive breath, as a sachet, and to scent face powders. HHRM p. 159.

OSIER, RED **Cornaceæ**

(RED OSIER DOGWOOD, SWAMP DOGWOOD, SILKY CORNEL)

Cornus sericea

Astringent, tonic, and stimulant; valuable in dyspepsia, diarrhea, diseases of the uterus, and to check the vomiting so common to pregnancy. When used in febrile diseases, it strengthens the pulse.

OSWEGO TEA **Rustaceæ**

(SCARLET MONARDA, BEE BALM)

Monarda didyma, Monarda punctata

Rubefacient, stimulant, and carminative as well as aromatic.

PANSY HERB **Violaceæ**

(HEARTSEASE, WILD PANSY)

Viola tricolor

Acts gently on the bowels, kidneys, and heart. Much used in ointments for skin diseases, including eczema and scald-head. HHRM p. 204.

PAREIRA BRAVA **Menispermaceæ**

(VELVET LEAF, ICE VINE)

Chondrodendron tomentosum

Tonic, diuretic, and aperient; one of the most valuable remedies for inflammation of the urinary passages, kidneys, and bladder; used in cases of gravel or calculus. Also recommended for dropsy, leucorrhoea, rheumatism, and jaundice.

PARSLEY LEAF **Umbelliferæ**

(PERSELY)

Apium petroselinum, Carum petroselinum, Petroselinum sativum

Either alone or combined with Cramp Bark, Black Haw, and Buchu, it will be found one of the best of remedies for female irregularities. It is excellent as a fomentation to cure bites and stings of insects. It is also a well-known article in culinary use. HHRM p. 141.

PARSLEY ROOT **Umbelliferæ**

(PERSELY)

Apium petroselinum, Carum petroselinum, Petroselinum sativum

A diuretic much esteemed in all dropsical affections, retention of the urine, and strangury. It is nutritive and much used in cooking. HHRM p. 141.

PARSLEY SEED **Umbelliferæ**

(PERSELY)

Apium petroselinum, Carum petroselinum, Petroselinum sativum

Carminative and tonic. A decoction of the crushed seeds, often in combination with Dill Seed is cooled and given to infants who suffer with colic and griping. HHRM p. 141.

PATCHOULI LEAVES **Labiatæ (Lamiaceæ)**

Pogostemon patchouli, Pogostemon cablin

A perfume agent; it acts as a moth repellent. HHRM p. 142.

PEACH TREE LEAVES **Rosaceæ**

Amygdalis persica, Persica vulgaris, Prunus persica

A mild laxative; exerts a sedative influence over the nervous system. Used with good results for whooping cough, irritable bladder and urethra, and inflammation of the stomach. Good as a hair tonic, too. HHRM p. 143.

PENNYROYAL **Labiatæ**

Mentha pulegium

Relieves colic and intestinal gas. Promotes perspiration, restores suppressed lochia, and is excellent in exciting the menstrual discharge. HHRM p. 143.

PEONY ROOT **Ranunculaceæ**

Pæonia officinalis

Highly esteemed as a remedy for epilepsy and to relieve internal pains, also valuable in spasms, nervous diseases, and whooping cough. HHRM p. 144.

PEPPERGRASS **Cruciferæ**

(SHEPHERD'S PURSE, LADY'S PURSE, PEPPER-AND-SALT)

Capsella bursa-pastoris, Lepidium virginicum

Remedies bleeding from the stomach, lungs, and kidneys; prescribed when blood or mucus is found in the urine. Anti-scorbutic. Soothing to Poison Ivy or Poison Oak blisters. Excellent in hair tonics. *Illustration: p. 68.*

PEPPERMINT **Labiatæ**

Mentha piperita

A valued remedy for wind colic, chills and fever; allays nausea, vomiting, coughs, and spasms. A topical anodyne. A refreshing tea. HHRM p. 134.

PEPPER, BLACK **Piperaceæ**

Piper nigrum

A digestive aid and stimulant with many culinary uses. It is often taken as a tea with Lemon and honey for colds. HHRM p. 52.

PEPPER, RED **Solanaceæ**

(AFRICAN BIRD PEPPER, CAPSICUM, CAYENNE PEPPER, CHILI PEPPER)

Capsicum annum

A powerful stimulant and anodyne, used in colds, rheumatism, spasmodic affections, and cholera. It is also a culinary staple. HHRM p. 166.

PERUVIAN BARK **Rubiaceæ**

(CHINCHONA, JESUITS' BARK, RED BARK)

Cinchona officinalis

Very valuable in all febrile, eruptive, and inflammatory diseases of a periodic nature. In general debility, it is a superior bitter tonic and astringent. Used as a gargle and in toothpaste to tighten the gums.

PICHI TOPS **Solanaceæ**

(FABIANA)

Fabiana imbricata

Diuretic. Helpful in the removal of kidney gravel and in cases of cystitis.

PILEWORT **Ranunculaceæ**

(FIGWORT, SMALLWORT, LESSER CELANDINE)

Ranunculus ficaria

As the name indicates, as an ointment or poultice, it is a remedy for piles.

PINK ROOT **Loganiaceæ**

(INDIAN PINK, MARYLAND PINK, WORMGRASS, STARBLOOM)

Spigelia marylandica

An active and certain vermifuge, the standard remedy for pin-worms; should be used in combination with Senna Leaves.

PIPSISSEWA **Ericaceæ**

(WINTER GREEN, BUTTER WINTER, PRINCE'S PINE, KING'S CURE, GROUND HOLLY, LOVE IN WINTER, RHEUMATISM WEED)

Chimaphila umbellata, Pyrola umbellata

Very useful in scrofula, chronic rheumatism, gonorrhea, strangury, kidney troubles, catarrh of the bladder and cutaneous diseases. *Illustration: p. 73.*

PLANTAIN LEAVES **Plantaginaceæ**

(RIPPLE GRASS, WAYBREAD, SNAKEWEED, WHITE MAN'S FOOT)

Plantago major

Beneficial in bacterial diseases, leucorrhoea, and diarrhea. Makes a soothing, cooling, and healing application in cases of ulcers and sores. The fresh juice and seeds are useful in cases of cough and vomiting; also prized by many mothers as a cure for bed wetting in children. The large, flat leaves are used to bind wounds. HHRM p. 156, *146*.

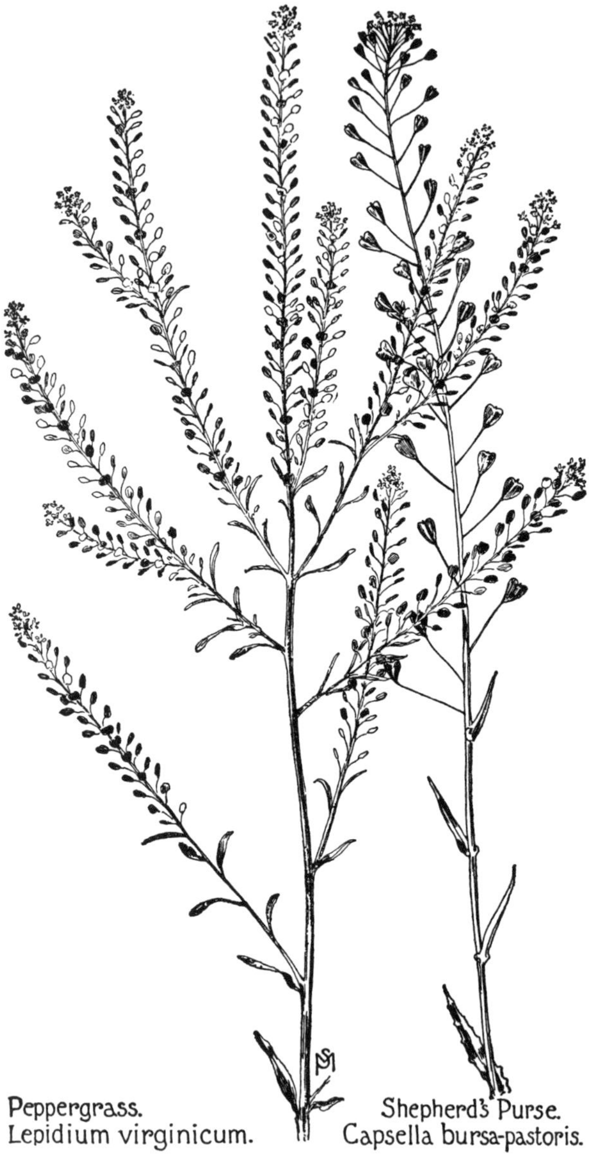

11. **Peppergrass**, *page 66.*

PLEURISY ROOT **Asclepiadaceæ**

(BUTTERFLY-WEED, SWALLOW-WORT, TUBER ROOT, WIND ROOT, COLIC ROOT, ORANGE MILKWEED)

Asclepias tuberosa

Expectorant, anti-spasmodic, and anodyne. Highly esteemed for bronchitis, pleurisy, fevers, breaking up colds, and treating catarrh of the lungs. Also used for flatulency, colic, indigestion, and acute rheumatism. HHRM p. 61.

POKE ROOT **Phytolaccaceæ**

(POKE BERRY ROOT)

Phytolacca americana, Phytolacca decandra

Emetic, purgative, and narcotic. An overdose may lead to convulsions and death. Notwithstanding, the young spring shoots, called Poke Salad, are eaten in moderation to purify the blood and may benefit cases of syphilis, scrofula, and similar bacterial blood and skin diseases. As an ointment, it is used to treat chronic rheumatism and piles. HHRM p. 156.

POMEGRANATE **Lythraceæ**

(GRENADIER)

Punica granatum

The rind is valuable in leucorrhea and female complaints; also, good in cases of night sweats, and intermittent fevers, The bark is a recognized remedy of great merit for worms; much used in combination with Pink Root and Senna. The seeds and juice find culinary favour.

POPLAR BARK **Salicaceæ**

(AMERICAN ASPEN, WHITE POPLAR, QUAKING ASPEN)

Populus tremuloides

Used with good results in emaciation and debility, impaired digestion, chronic diarrhea, intermittent fever, kidney and rheumatic complaints, liver troubles, gallstones, jaundice, and worms.

PRIMROSE FLOWERS **Primulaceæ**

(COWSLIP)

Primula officinalis, Primula vulgaris, Primula veris

Anti-spasmodic, astringent, and expectorant. Useful in nervous hysteria, nervous headaches, and muscular rheumatism. The whole plant is sedative; in higher doses it is emetic. HHRM p. 158.

PRIVET **Oleaceæ**

Ligustrum vulgare, Ligustrum ovalifolium

This is astringent. Valued in bowel complaints, ulcerations of the stomach and bowels, or as a gargle for ulcers and eruptions of the mouth and throat.

PSYLLIUM SEEDS **Plantaginaceæ**

(PSYLLIUM PLANTAIN, FLEASEED, PSYLLION, PSYLLIOS)

Plantago psyllium

A sovereign drugless laxative. It relieves constipation and as an internal lubricant it is far superior to mineral oil. It has nutritive value and can be baked into pleasing foods that act as an effective bowel regulator that is easily tolerated by costive children.

PUMPKIN SEEDS **Cucurbitacea**

Cucurbita pepo

A favourite and easily tolerated vermifuge. Also of nutritive value.

PYROLA **Ericaceæ (Pyrolaceæ)**

(YEVERING BELLS, PINK WINTERGREEN)

Pyrola secunda, Pyrola asarifolia

Astringent, diuretic, tonic, and anti-spasmodic.

QUASSIA **Simaroubaceæ**

(BITTER ASH, BITTER WOOD, BITTER ROOT)

Quassia amara, Picrænia excelsa

Similar to Simaruba, and likewise used in rheumatism, remittent and intermittent fevers, dyspepsia, and debility. Additionally, it is employed to destroy the appetite for alcoholic drinks. It is an insecticide; a strong tea sprayed on aphid-infested vegetables will protect them from depredation. It is also used to destroy human parasites such as lice, scabies, fleas, pin-worms, and mosquitoes, and to stop rosacea flare-ups. HHRM p. 159.

QUINCE SEED **Rosaceæ**

(GOLDEN APPLE)

Cydonia vulgaris, Pyrus cydonia

Demulcent and mucilaginous. Useful in diarrhea, dysentery, sore mouth, and as a wash for inflamed and sore eyes. Also much used as a means of keeping the hair in curl. HHRM p. 161.

RAGGED CUP **Compositæ**

(INDIAN CUP PLANT, RAGGED CUP)

Silphium perfoliatum

Tonic, diaphoretic, and alterative. Freshens the breath and prevents nausea and vomiting; also useful for cough and asthma. The young leaves may be eaten as salad.

RAGWORT **Compositæ**

(SATYRION, STINKING NANNY, STAMMERWORT, CUSHAG)

Senecio jacobæa, Jacobæa vulgaris

Detergent, stimulant, and astringent. A reputed aphrodisiac.

RED OAK BARK **Fagaceæ**

(NORTHERN RED OAK, CHAMPION OAK)

Quercus rubra

Very highly prized as a douche for leucorrhea and female genital troubles. Used also in sore throat, offensive ulcers, obstinate chronic diarrhea, hemorrhage, and as a gargle or injection in piles.

RED RASPBERRY LEAVES **Rosaceæ**

(RASPBIS, HINDBERRY, BRAMBLE OF MOUNT IDA)

Rubus idæus, Rubus occidentalis, Rubus odoratus, Rubus strigosus

Good for sick stomach and vomiting and very efficient in cases of diarrhea, dysentery, cholera, hemorrhage from the stomach or bowels, or uterine flooding. Utilized as a vaginal douche in cases of leucorrhea and genital canker. *Illustration: p. 78.* HHRM p. 162.

RED ROOT **Rhamnaceæ**

(NEW JERSEY TEA, WILD SNOWBALL)

Ceanothus americanus

Used with great good effect in dysentery, gonorrhea, asthma, chronic bronchitis, whooping cough, and consumption; also as a gargle in cases of canker and sore mouth.

RED SAUNDERS **Leguminosæ**

(RED SANTAL, RED SANDALWOOD, RUBYWOOD, SAPPAN)

Pterocarpus santalinus, Pterocarpi lignum, Santalum rubrum

Astringent; also used as a colouring agent for tinctures and in incense.

RHATANY **Polygalaceæ**

(KRAMERIA, MAPATO, PERUVIAN RHATANY, RED RHATANY)

Krameria triandra

An old and reliable remedy for chronic diarrhea and dysentery; also excellent for incontinence of the urine, leucorrhea, profuse menstruation, hemorrhages, vomiting of blood, spongy gums, and canker.

RHUBARB ROOT **Polygonaceeæ**

(ENGLISH RHUBARB, CHINESE RHUBARB)

Rheum officinale, Rheum palmatum, Rheum rhaponticum

Cathartic, astringent and tonic; extensively used as a purgative and in chronic diarrhea, dysentery, convalescence from exhausting diseases when a mild cathartic is required, infantile complaints, dyspepsia, and headaches.

ROCK BRAKE **Filices**

(WALL FERN, BRAKE ROOT, OAK FERN)

Polypodium vulgare

Efficacious in diarrhea, night sweats, to remove worms, and as an injection for leucorrhea and suppression of the lochia. Much used for lame back caused by kidney and bladder troubles, also for dry cough. HHRM p. 93.

ROMAN MOTHERWORT **Labiatæ**

(MOTHERWORT)

Leonurus cardiaca

Universally used to relieve suppression of the menses or lochia, and in other female complaints. Good for nervousness, delirium, wakefulness, disturbed sleep, colds, gallstones, and liver troubles. HHRM p. 135, *122.*

ROSE **Rosaceæ**

Rosa spp.

The fruits, called hips, are anti-scorbutic. The petals are tonic and mildly astringent; with Sassafras pith they make a soothing application for sore and inflamed eyes and are excellent as a mouth wash. HHRM p. 168.

ROSEMARY **Labiatæ**

Rosmarinus officinalis

An effective remedy for female complaints. The warm infusion is taken for colds, colic, and nervous conditions. A notable hair tonic. HHRM p. 169.

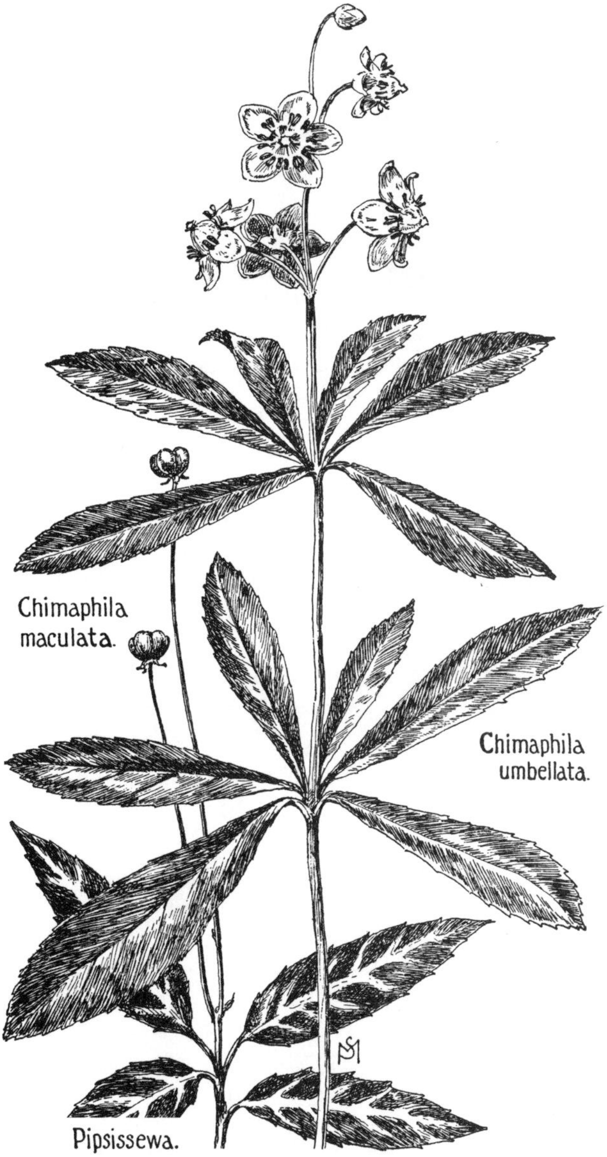

12. **Pipsissewa**, *page 67.*

RUE **Rutaceæ**

(RUTA, RUDA)

Ruta graveolens

A common remedy for worms, flatulent colic, hysterics, and epilepsy; also effective in overcoming suppression of the menses. It may also be applied as a poultice to sore or inflamed eyes. HHRM p. 170.

RUPTURE WORT **Caryophyllaceæ**

(SMOOTH RUPTUREWORT)

Herniaria glabra

Diuretic used in cystitis, as well as cardiac or nephritic dropsy. As a mild astringent it finds use in ophthalmic cases as an eye wash.

SAFFRON **Iridaceæ**

(SPANISH SAFFRON)

Crocus sativus

One of the most reliable remedies in cases of measles and other eruptive diseases; also beneficial in regulating the menstrual discharge and in iron deficiency anemia or chlorosis hysteria of young women. HHRM p. 172.

SAGE **Labiatæ**

(SALVIA)

Salvia officinalis, Salvia spp.

Highly esteemed for dyspepsia and stomach troubles; also valuable as a vermifuge, to produce perspiration, and as a gargle for sore throat. Used in scalp tonics. A pleasant seasoning for meats and poultry. HHRM p. 172.

SAINT JOHN'S BREAD **Leguminosæ**

(LOCUST PODS, CAROB, SUGAR PODS)

Ceratonia siliqua

Used as a laxative and a flavouring agent; it remotely resembles Cocoa.

SAINT JOHN'S WORT **Hypericaceæ**

(HYPERICUM)

Hypericum perforatum, Hypericum ellipticum

Highly prized for purifying the blood, also used in suppression of the urine, chronic urinary affections, diarrhea, dysentery, worms, jaundice, and to regulate the menstrual discharge and relieve female troubles.

SALEP **Orchidaceæ**

(ADAM AND EVE ROOT, PUTTY ROOT ORCHID, SALOOP ROOT)

Aplectrum hyemale, Orchis mascula, Orchis morio, Orchis militaris, Orchis ustulata, Orchis coriophora, etc.

Used as a demulcent. It is also nutritive. HHRM p. 19.

SANDALWOOD **Santalaceæ**

Santalum album

Promotes perspiration and is an agreeable stimulant. It is much used to place in storage boxes and drawers, because of its fragrance. It may also be burned as an incense, HHRM p. 178.

SARSAPARILLA **Liliaceæ**

(SASPARILLA, CHANEY ROOT, CHAINEY ROOT)

Smilax officinalis, Smilax medica, Smilax sarsaparilla, Smilax regelii, Smilax balbisiana

A most highly extolled blood purifier, used in chronic diseases of the skin, venereal complaints, dropsy, rheumatic affections, and all cases where a good alterative is required. HHRM p. 178, *146*.

SASSAFRAS **Lauraceæ**

Sassafras officinale

The bark is a warm and agreeable tonic for stomach and bowels; valuable in wind and colic, eruptive diseases, and as a flavour corrective for other medicines. The pith is much used as an eye wash in ophthalmia or inflammation of the eyes. HHRM p. 179.

SAVIN **Coniferæ**

(SAVINE TOPS)

Sabina cacumina

Highly recommended for chronic rheumatism, also for obstructed menstruation, suppression of urine, and other kidney complaints.

SAW PALMETTO **Palmaceæ**

(SABAL)

Sarenoa serrulata

Of great service in chronic bronchitis, asthma, cold in the head, whooping cough, and irritated mucous membranes of the throat and nose. A genito-urinary antiseptic and sedative in all diseases of the reproductive organs.

SAXIFRAGE **Umbelliferæ**

(PIMPINELLA, LESSER BURNET)

Pimpinella saxifraga

Aromatic, stomachic, diaphoretic, and diuretic. Also used as a gargle to relieve a hoarse throat. Used as a substitute for Anise. HHRM p. 31.

SCABISH **Onagraceæ**

(COMMON EVENING-PRIMROSE, TEA PRIMROSE)

Oenothera biennis

Highly prized as a remedy for tetter, salt rheum, and other skin diseases and eruptions, also for cough.

SCULLCAP **Labiatæ**

(SKULLCAP, HELMET FLOWER, HOODWORT)

Scutellaria galericulata, Scutellaria minor, Scutellaria lateriflora

Astringent, anti-spasmodic, anti-inflammatory, mildly anodyne. A favourite nerve tonic, valued in nervous complaints, including wakefulness, delirium tremens, convulsions, excitability, and neuralgia. When chewed, it soothes toothache. It has also been found useful in epilepsy. HHRM p. 185, *171.*

SEA WRACK **Fucaceæ**

(BLADDER WRACK, FUCUS, BLASENTANG, SEETANG)

Fucus vesiculosis, Fucus vesiculeux

An unsurpassed remedy for obesity, also good in case of scrofula, goiter, and all glandular affections; acts on the kidneys and relieves that distressing feeling of "stuffiness." Has a tonic effect in many cases.

SENECA SNAKE ROOT **Polygalaceæ**

(MILKWORT, SENEGA SNAKEROOT, RATTLESNAKE ROOT)

Polygala senega

Esteemed highly for affections of the lungs, croup, coughs, chronic catarrh, and asthma; use with Blood Root and Pleurisy Root. HHRM p. 181, *122.*

SENNA LEAVES **Leguminosæ (Fabaceæ)**

(CASSIA, CASSIA SENNA)

Cassia acutifolia, Cassia angustifolia, Cassia marilandica, Senna alexandrina

A valuable cathartic, mild and effectual, excellent for bilious complaints, bad taste in the mouth, worms and the like. HHRM p. 181.

SHEEP SORREL **Polygonaceæ**

(FIELD SORREL)

Rumex acetosella

Used in scurvy, scrofula and skin diseases, and as a poultice for wens, boils and tumours. It is reputed to cure cancer.

SILVER WEED **Rosaceæ**

(SILVERY CINQUEFOIL, POTENTILLA, FIVE-FINGER GRASS)

Potentilla anserina

Aromatic, bitter, astringent, tonic, and febrifuge. A remedy for cramping in the stomach and bowels. Drinking the tea and accompanying this by a sitting-bath in a stronger infusion will check bleeding piles. The tea is also recommended in jaundice and malarial fevers. HHRM p. 95, *23.*

SIMARUBA **Simarubaceæ**

(DYSENTERY BARK)

Simaruba amara, Simaruba officinalis, Simarouba excelsa

A bitter tonic, similar to Quassia, esteemed as a restorative in the later stages of dysentery; it builds up intestinal tone and acts as a mild sedative for the debilitated patient. The dose must be monitored because in excess, it can produce vomiting, thus undoing the good it has accomplished.

SKUNK CABBAGE **Araceæ**

(POLE CAT WEED)

Symplocarpus fœtidus

Successfully used in whooping cough, asthma, rheumatism, convulsions, spasms, hysteria, and nervous irritability. *Illustration: p. 78.* HHRM p. 185.

SOAP BARK **Rosaceæ**

(PANAMA BARK, CULLAY, QUILLAJA BARK)

Quillaja saponaria

Expectorant; stimulates mucus. Used in shampoo preparations for the hair.

SOLOMON'S SEAL **Liliaceæ**

Convallaria polygonatum, Convallaria multiflorum, Polygonatum biflora, etc.

Prized highly as a remedy for female complaints, leucorrhea, piles, pectoral affections, erysipelas, and as a wash for Poison Ivy, Poison Oak, insect bites. and other inflamed surfaces. HHRM p. 188, *171.*

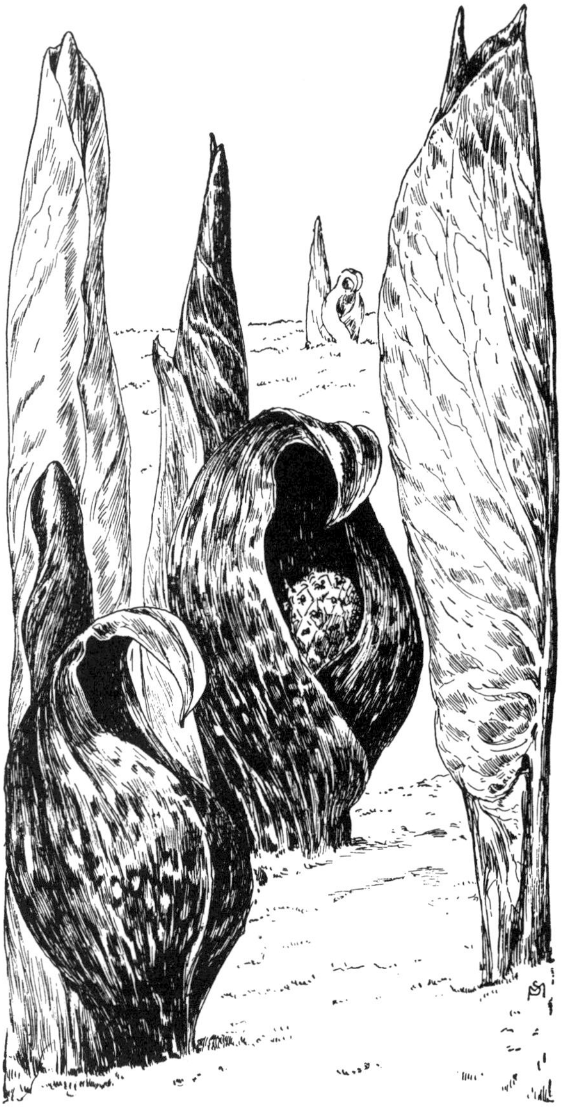

Skunk Cabbage. Symplocarpus fœtidus.

13. **Skunk Cabbage**, *page 77.*

SOUTHERNWOOD **Compositæ**

(OLD MAN, LAD'S LOVE)

Artemisia abrotanum

An agreeable bitter tonic for dyspepsia, indigestion, and wind in the stomach; valuable in obstructions and to remove worms. HHRM p. 190.

SPEARMINT **Labiatæ**

(GARDEN MINT, GREEN MINT, SPIRE MINT, LAMB MINT)

Mentha viridis, Mentha spicata

One of the best remedies for colic, wind in the bowels, and dyspepsia. Valuable to prevent vomiting, in spasms, dropsy, gravel suppression, or scalding urine, and as a local application for piles. HHRM p. 134.

SPEEDWELL **Scrophulariaceæ**

(VERONICA)

Veronica officinalis

Tonic, alterative and diuretic; used with good results in asthma and coughs.

SPIKENARD **Compositæ**

(PLOUGHMAN'S SPIKENARD)

Inula conyza

Good for skin itch, pimples, or wounds when combined with Burdock, Yellow Dock, and Barberry. Also used in coughs, colds, and pulmonary affections. A help in pregnancy and parturition. HHRM p. 191.

SQUAW VINE **Rubiaceæ**

(PARTRIDGEBERRY, CHECKERBERRY)

Mitchellia repens

One of the best remedies for female complaints; a powerful uterine tonic. Highly beneficial after parturition for suppression of the lochia. Also diuretic; used in cases of dropsy and suppression of urine. HHRM p. 192.

STAR ANISE **Magnoliaceæ**

(ANISE ESTRELLA, BADIANA, CHINESE ANISE)

Illicium verum

Stimulant and carminative; used in cases of flatulence, colic in infants, and to remove nausea. Sometimes added to other medicines to improve their flavour or to correct disagreeable effects. HHRM p. 192.

STILLINGIA **Euphorbiaceæ**

(QUEEN'S ROOT, QUEEN'S DELIGHT, SILVER LEAF, YAW ROOT)

Stillingia sylvatica, Sapium sylvaticum

One of the meat valuable remedies for scrofula and skin diseases, as well as for chronic affections of the liver. Also highly esteemed for bronchitis, laryngitis, and all lung complaints. HHRM p. 160.

STONE ROOT **Labiatæ**

(HORSEWEED, RICHWEED, KNOB-ROOT, OXBALM, KNOT-ROOT)

Collinsonia canadensis

Very useful in chronic catarrh of the bladder, leucorrhoea. kidney gravel, and dropsy; also of value for chronic debility of the stomach, and similar ailments.

STRAWBERRY LEAVES **Rosaceæ**

(GARDEN STRAWBERRY, FRAGARIA, WILD STRAWBERRY)

Fragaria vesca, Fragaria virginiana

Much prized for dysentery, diarrhea, intestinal debility, and night sweats; also good for the appetite. *Illustration: p. 83.*

SUMAC BARK **Anacardiaceæ**

(SUMACH, SHOEMAKE)

Rhus copalina, Rhus glabrum, Rhus typhina, Rhus hirta

Valuable in gonorrhea, leucorrhea, hectic fever, and scrofula, cleansing to the entire system. HHRM p. 194, *197.*

SUMAC BERRIES **Anacardiaceæ**

(SUMACH, SHOEMAKE)

Rhus copalina, Rhus glabrum, Rhus typhina, Rhus hirta

Highly esteemed for bowel complaints, diabetes, and febrile diseases. For mouth canker and sore mouth it has no superior. HHRM p. 194.

SUMBUL **Umbelliferæ**

(EURYANGIUM MUSK ROOT, JATAMANSI, OUCHI)

Ferula sumbul

Anti-spasmodic, useful in epilepsy, asthma, delirium tremens, hysteria, and female nervousness, especially when combined with Valerian. Also useful in amenorrhea, chlorosis, leucorrhea, and gleet.

SUMMER SAVORY **Labiatæ**

(BOHNENKRAUT)

Satureia hortensis

Very beneficial in colds, menstrual suppression, and as a gentle stimulating tonic after fevers. A warm, agreeable remedy for wind colic and dyspepsia. Used with Sage as a seasoning for sausage, meat, and poultry dressing.

SUNDEW **Droseraceæ**

(DEW PLANT, ROUND-LEAVED SUNDEW, RED ROT)

Drosera rotundifolia

This herb has long been esteemed as a remedy for chronic bronchitis, asthma, and whooping cough.

SUNFLOWER SEEDS **Compositæ**

(MARIGOLD OF PERU, CORONA SOLIS, SOLA INDIANUS)

Helianthus annuus, Chrysanthemum peruvianum

Much used in coughs and pulmonary affections, also in dysentery and inflammation of the bladder and kidneys. Nutritive.

SWEET FERN **Umbelliferæ**

(SWEET CHERVIL, SWEET CICELY, COW CHERVIL)

Myrrhis odorata

Aromatic, stomachic, carminative, and expectorant, resembling Anise. Very effective in dysentery, leucorrhea, bruises, and debility after fevers.

SWEET FLAG **Araceæ**

(CALAMUS)

Acorus calamus

A good remedy for wind colic and internals pains, and useful to prevent the griping of other medicines. Excellent for dyspepsia, feeble digestion, and to aid the action of Peruvian Bark in intermittent fevers. HHRM p. 63, *71*.

SWEET GUM **Hamamelidaceæ**

(LIQUIDAMBAR, STORAX)

Liquidambar orientalis, Liquidambar styraciflua

As a remedy for catarrh, coughs, and pulmonary affections generally, it is without an equal. It is also very valuable for fever sores and scrofula, when made into an ointment. HHRM p. 195.

TAMARACK BARK **Pinaceæ**

(HACKMATACK, EASTERN LARCH, BLACK LARCH, RED LARCH)

Larix laricina

A good remedy for rheumatism. It is used for increasing the appetite and purifying the blood; also recommended for jaundice, gallstones, and obstructions of the liver.

TANSY **Compositæ**

(GOLDEN BUTTONS)

Tanecetum vulgare

One of the most popular remedies for promoting the menstrual flow; also good for fever and ague, dropsy, worms, hysterics, and as a fomentation in swellings and tumours. HHRM p. 196.

TARRAGON **Compositæ**

(LITTLE DRAGON, ESTRAGON, FRENCH TARRAGON)

Artemisia dracunculus

Fragrant and stimulating to the appetite, hence it is used for seasoning purposes.

THISTLE, BLESSED **Compositæ**

(HOLY THISTLE)

Carbenia benedicta, Carduus benedictus, Cnicus benedictus

Tonic and diaphoretic. Taken cold in a mild dose, it is gentle tonic in debility of the stomach. HHRM p. 54.

THYME **Labiatæ**

Thymus vulgaris, Thymus serpyllum

Used with good results in painful or obstructed menstruation, also for internal pain in the bladder, good for dyspepsia, weak stomach, hysteria, flatulence, colic, headache, and to produce perspiration. HHRM p. 198.

TOAD FLAX **Scrophulariaceæ**

(BUTTER-AND-EGGS, SNAPDRAGON, DEVIL'S HEAD, EGGS AND BACON, MONKEY FLOWER)

Linaria vulgaris, Linaria canadensis

Diuretic and in higher doses cathartic; has been used in dropsy, jaundice, and cutaneous eruptions. *Illustration: p. 88.*

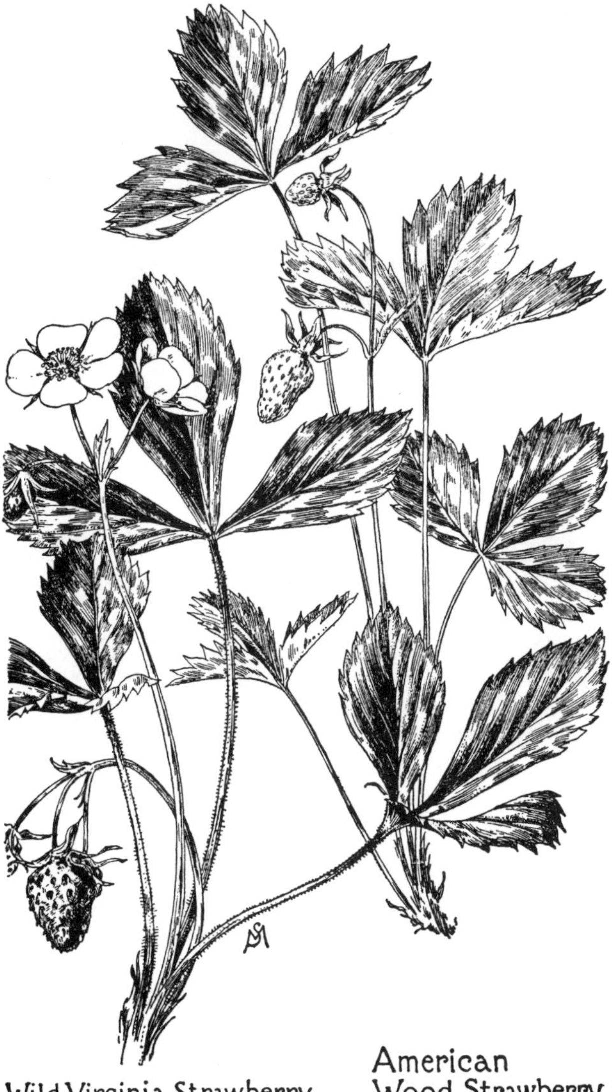

14. **Strawberry Leaves**, *page 80.*

TURKEY CORN **Furnariaceæ**

(SQUIRREL CORN, BLEEDING HEART, CORYDALIS)

Dicentra canadensis, Corydalis canadensis, Bicuculla canadensis

Much prized as a remedy for scrofula and skin diseases.

TURMERIC **Zingiberaceæ**

(YELLOW GINGER)

Curcuma longa

A fragrant, aromatic stimulant and excitant, after the manner of Ginger and Zedoary. It is used in cooking for its flavour and attractive yellow colour.

TWIN LEAF **Berberidaceæ**

(JEFFERSONIA, RHEUMATISM ROOT)

Jeffersonia diphylla

Used in chronic rheumatism, dropsy, nervous affections, cramps, and spasms; also as a gargle in throat troubles, scarlatina, and indolent ulcers.

UNICORN ROOT **Liliaceæ**

(AGUE ROOT, BETTIE GRASS, DEVIL'S BIT, STAR ROOT, STAR GRASS)

Aletris farinosa

A valuable bitter stomachic and one of the best remedies for imparting tone and vigour to the bladder. It greatly strengthens the female generative organs, affording protection against miscarriage, and acts as an excellent remedy for falling of the womb. HHRM p. 200.

UVA-URSI LEAVES **Ericaceæ**

(BEARBERRY, KINNIKINNICK, UPLAND CRANBERRY)

Arctostaphylos officinalis, Arctostaphylos uva-ursi

Used in all affections of the kidneys, bladder, and urinary passages, cystitis, strangury, and mucous discharges with the urine. HHRM p. 45, *23*.

VALERIAN **Valerianacæ**

(VANDAL ROOT)

Valeriana officinalis, Valeriana sylvatica, Valeriana uliginosa

Anodyne; eases and quiets pain, producing a gentle sleep; invaluable in chorea, nervous debility, hysteria, and low forms of fever where a nervous stimulant is required. HHRM p. 201.

VANILLA PODS **Orchidaceæ**

Vanilla planifolia

An aromatic stimulant, it is used in infusion in hysteria, rheumatism, and low forms of fever. It is also called an aphrodisiac, and it said to be powerfully exciting to the generative system. HHRM p. 201.

VERVAIN **Verbenaceæ**

(VERBENA)

Verbena officinalis

Much used for its quieting and easing effect, also considered valuable in cases of female complaints, obstructed menses, intermittent fevers, colds, gravel, and worms; externally it is very healing to sores. HHRM p. 202.

VIOLET FLOWERS **Violaceæ**

(HEARTSEASE, SWEET VIOLET, VIOLA)

Viola odorata, Viola blanda, Viola sagittata, Viola ovata, etc.

Expectorant and, in larger doses, emetic. HHRM p. 204, *197.*

VIOLET LEAVES **Violaceæ**

(HEARTSEASE, SWEET VIOLET, VIOLA)

Viola odorata, Viola blanda, Viola sagittata, Viola ovata, etc.

An excellent soothing and healing remedy for inflammation of the stomach and bowels; good for skin diseases, especially when combined with Red Clover; also used for coughs, colds, and sore throat. HHRM p. 204, *197.*

VIRGINIA SNAKE ROOT **Aristolochiaceæ**

Aristolochia serpentaria

An excellent blood purifier, much used in cases of skin diseases and fevers. Often combined with Yellow Dock and Sarsaparilla as a Spring tonic. Produces perspiration, strengthens the stomach, and increases the appetite; also good in rheumatic complaints. HHRM p. 204, *197.*

WAHOO **Celastraceæ**

(WA'AHOO, BURNING BUSH)

Euonymus americanus, Euonymus atropurpureus

Enjoys a great reputation as a sovereign remedy for dropsy; also a good and effective laxative, and very useful in intermittent fevers, dyspepsia, torpid liver, and pulmonary affections. HHRM p. 205.

WALNUT HULL **Juglandaceæ**

(BLACK WALNUT, ENGLISH WALNUT, PERSIAN WALNUT)

Juglans nigra, Juglans regia

Hulls of the nuts are used in a dye for the hair, for making dark brown ink, and for tanning or dyeing leather and cloth. HHRM p. 205.

WALNUT LEAVES **Juglandaceæ**

(BLACK WALNUT, ENGLISH WALNUT, PERSIAN WALNUT)

Juglans nigra, Juglans regia

Alterative, laxative, and astringent; an excellent bowel and liver regulator, a good remedy for anemia and jaundice; useful for herpes and eczema. The leaves are also repellent to many species of insects. HHRM p. 205.

WATER ERYNGO **Umbelliferæ**

(CORN SNAKE ROOT, ERYNGOES, RATTLESNAKE CONQUEROR, RATTLESNAKE MASTER, SEA HOLLY, SEA HOLM)

Eryngium aquaticum, Eryngium campestre, Eryngium fœtidum, Eryngium maritimum, Eryngium virginianum, Eryngium yuccefolium

Aphrodisiac, exciting venereal desires, also diuretic, stimulant, diaphoretic, expectorant, and, in large doses, emetic. HHRM p. 164.

WATER PEPPER **Polygonacæ**

(SMART WEED)

Polygonum hydropiperoides, Polygonum punctatum

Used with good results in uterine diseases and disorders, also amenorrhea, gravel, colds, coughs, bowel complaints, erysipelas. HHRM p. 185, *171.*

WHITE HOLLY LEAVES **Aquifoleaceæ**

(HOLM, HOLLY, HOLY TREE)

Ilex aquifolium

Astringent, tonic, diaphoretic, diuretic, and alterative; a useful febrifuge in cases of catarrh and pleurisy; good for diarrhea and ulcers. HHRM p. 113.

WHITE OAK BARK **Cupuliferæ**

Quercus alba

A highly esteemed astringent, producing much the same effect as Red Oak. Especially valuable as a wash or injection for piles and internal sores of the lower bowels. HHRM p. 139.

WHITE PINE BARK — Pinaceæ

(WEYMOUTH PINE)

Pinus strobus, Pinus alba

An old reliable inhalant remedy for coughs and bronchial affections; also effectively used in rheumatism, and scurvy. A serviceable diuretic, it is held to be a valuable remedy in bladder, kidney, and urethral problems, as well as in diseases of the mucous membranes. Externally it is applied in the form of liniments or plasters. HHRM p. 155.

WHITE PINE NEEDLES — Pinaceæ

(WEYMOUTH PINE)

Pinus strobus, Pinus alba

This, in combination with Dog Grass, Althæa, Poplar Bark, and Uva-Ursi, gives an excellent remedy for dropsy and diabetes. HHRM p. 155.

WICKUP — Onagrariaceæ

(WILLOW-HERB, ROSE BAY, FLOWERING WILLOW, BLOOD VINE, BLOOMING SALLY, PURPLE ROCKET, WICOPY, TAME WITHY)

Epilobium angustifolium

It is excellent in dysentery or chronic diarrhea, or whenever an astringent is required; an effective tonic, soothing to inflammation, with anti-spasmodic properties helpful in whooping cough, hiccough, and asthma.

WILD GERANIUM — Geraniaceæ

(SPOTTED CRANESBILL, STORKSBILL, ALUM BLOOM, CROWFOOT)

Geranium maculatum

A powerful astringent and one of the best remedies for diarrhea, chronic dysentery, cholera infantum, and hemorrhage; also applied externally to stop bleeding. Produces sweating; improves the appetite, aids digestion, and promotes nutrition. For diarrhea in children, the decoction may given in milk, which covers the taste.

WILD SOAPWORT — Caryophyllaceæ

(SOAPROOT, BOUNCING BET, LATHERWORT, FULLER'S HERB, BRUISEWORT, CROW SOAP, SWEET BETTY)

Saponaria officinalis

Alterative and diaphoretic. It may be used as a substitute for soap in shampoo compounds. A decoction applied to the skin relieves itching.

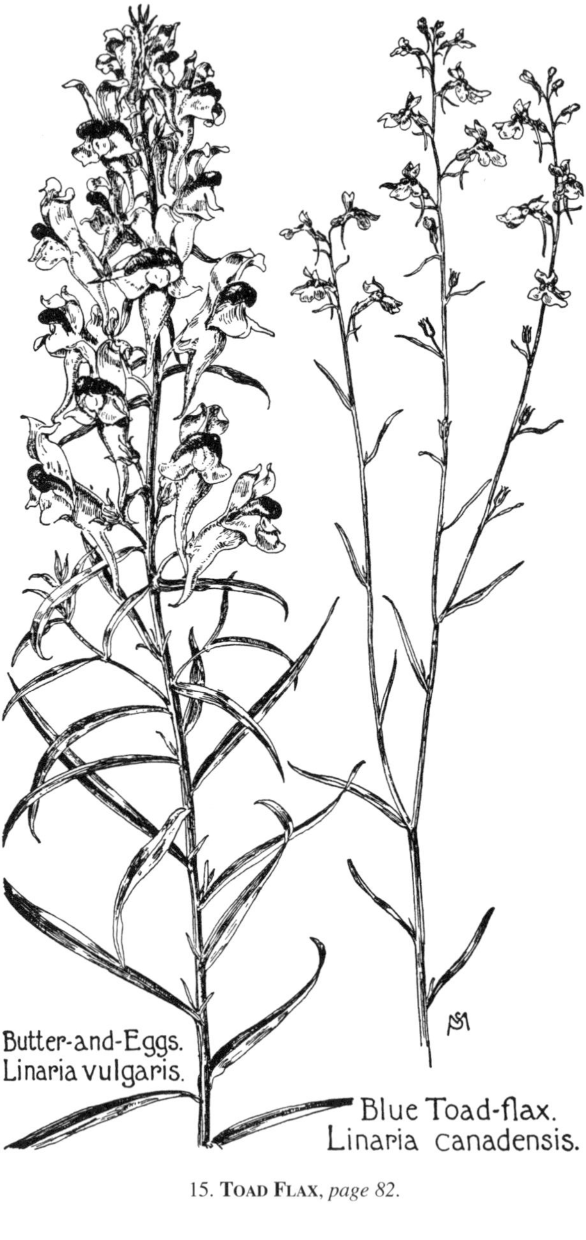

15. **Toad Flax**, *page 82*.

WILD YAM **Dioscoreaceæ**

(DIOSCOREA, COLIC ROOT, RHEUMATISM ROOT)

Dioscorea villosa

Very efficacious for bilious colic, gallstones, affections of the liver, spasms, rheumatism, and flatulency; also has a great reputation as a remedy for female complaints, including cramps and the afterpains of childbirth.

WILLOW BARK **Salicaceæ**

(WHITE WILLOW, EUROPEAN WILLOW)

Salix alba

Astringent, anodyne, and anti-inflammatory. Used in intermittent and periodic fevers, headache, debility of the digestive organs, diarrhea, dysentery, hemorrhages, and chronic mucous discharges. HHRM p. 206.

WINTERGREEN **Ericaceæ**

Gaultheria procumbens

For colic, upset stomach, and gas in the bowels, also valuable in dropsy. Small doses stimulate the heart, and are found to be useful in rheumatism and diabetes. Anti-inflammatory and anodyne; similar to Willow or aspirin. Has been used as a flavouring in toothpaste. HHRM p. 207.

WINTERS BARK **Magnoliaceæ**

(TRUE WINTER'S BARK, WINTER'S CINNAMON, WINTERA)

Drimys winteri

Stimulant, pungent, aromatic, and stomachic.

WITCH HAZEL BARK **Hamamelidaceæ**

(SPOTTED ALDER, WINTERBLOOM, SNAPPING HAZELNUT)

Hamamelis virginiana

One of the most highly prized remedies for external inflammation, as a wash for painful swellings, a gargle for canker, and injection for leucorrhea. Valuable in diarrhea, dysentery, and mucous discharges.

WOODRUFF **Rubiaceæ**

(SWEET WOODRUFF, MASTER OF THE WOODS, WOODS MASTER)

Asperula odorata

Of service as a liver corrective, a blood purifier, and aid to digestion. Keep with linens, like Lavender, to preserve them from insects. HHRM p. 133.

WOOD SORREL **Oxalidaceæ**

(WOOD SOUR, SOUR TREFOIL)

Oxalis acetosella

Cooling and diuretic, useful in febrile diseases hemorrhages, chronic catarrh, and urinary affections.

WORMSEED **Chenopodiaceæ**

(JERUSALEM OAK SEED, JESUIT'S TEA)

Chenopodium anthelminticum, Chenopodium ambrosiodes

One of the best remedies for expelling worms; a most valuable vermifuge; also very useful in the treatment of suppressed menses or amenorrhea.

WORMWOOD **Compositæ**

Artemisia absinthium

An old and always good remedy for bilious complaints, gallstones, liver troubles, jaundice, and intermittent fevers, highly esteemed to expel worms. Applied externally to bruises and sprains. HHRM p. 207.

YARROW **Compositæ**

(MILFOIL, SOLDIER'S WOUNDWORT, STAUNCHWEED)

Achillea millefolium

Most highly valued as a mildly anodyne vulnerary; it is also used to remediate hemorrhages and piles, and to restore continence of the urine. Useful in diabetes, dysentery, flatulence, as a douche in leucorrhea, and as a remedy for suppression of the menses. HHRM p. 208.

YELLOW BEARSFOOT **Compositæ**

(UVEDALIA, LEAF CUP, YELLOW LEAF CUP)

Polymnia uvedalia

Valued in rheumatism and arthritis, lumbago, and sciatica, as well as a febrifuge in rheumatic fever and malaria.

YELLOW DOCK **Polygonaceæ**

(CURLY DOCK)

Rumex crispus

One of the best of remedies for giving tone and strength to the system; highly valued in scrofula, diseases of eruptive nature and all cases where the blood needs purifying. Also used in ointments for itch. HHRM p. 208.

YELLOW PARILLA **Menispermaceæ**

(CANADIAN MOONSEED, TEXAS SARSAPARILLA, MOONSEED SARSAPARILLA, VINE MAPLE)

Menispermum canadense

An old standby for an appetizer and general all-around tonic, a superior laxative bitter; used in scrofula, gout, rheumatism, and cutaneous diseases.

YELLOWROOT **Ranunculaceæ**

Xanthorhiza simplicissima

A pure bitter tonic; reputed to be useful in mouth infections and sore throat.

YERBA MANSA **Saururaceæ**

(LIZARD TAIL)

Anemopsis californica

Peppery and astringent, it is chewed to bring relief to troubles of the mucous membranes, and can be applied outwardly for rheumatic pains.

YERBA REUMA **Frankeniaceæ**

(PALMER'S SEA-HEATH, PALMER'S FRANKENIA)

Frankenia palmeri

Useful in treating nasal catarrh, catarrhal gonorrhea, and leucorrhea.

YERBA SANTA **Hydrophyllaceæ**

(HOLY HERB, SACRED HERB)

Eriodictyon californicum, Eriodictyon glutinosum, Eriodictyon tomentosum

Considered very valuable in affections of the lungs, chronic laryngitis and bronchitis, nasal catarrh, and rheumatism. HHRM p. 208.

YOHIMBE **Rubiaceæ**

(JOHIMBE)

Pausinystalia johimbe

Stimulant aphrodisiac; corrects sexual troubles and difficulties.

ZEDOARY **Zingiberaceæ**

(WHITE TURMERIC)

Curcuma zedoaria

Carminative and stomachic, it is also an excellent anti-inflammatory and vulnerary. It eases pain, and remediates menstrual irregularities.

HOW TO MAKE AND USE HERBAL MEDICINES

- **Tea or Infusion:** Place a heaping teaspoonful of your herb or herbs in a cup. Fill the cup with boiling water, cover, and let stand until cool enough to drink. This is called "steeping." Drink the liquid only, not the herbs.
- **Decoction:** For woody roots or barks, make a decoction made by boiling the material for several minutes. Drink the liquid only, not the herbs.
- **Bath or Wash:** After making your infusion or a decoction, simply dilute the liquid and use it as a sitting-bath, foot-soak, or topical application.
- **Steeping bag:** When making infusions, decoctions, or baths, you may employ a muslin bag to hold the herbs. After removing the bag from the liquid, turn it inside-out, rinse it, and let it dry. It will last for many uses.
- **Tincture:** Steep tightly-packed herbs in brandy or whiskey. After two weeks, remove the herbs. The usual dosage is a teaspoonful. For a stronger tincture, repeat the process with a second or third "run" of herbs.
- **Ointment:** A simple ointment can be made with unsalted butter or lard. Melt it, pour it over the herbs to cover, let the mixture sit one week, melt again, and strain off the herbs. Repeat for at least three "runs" of herbs. Add a small amount of beeswax at the end to make a firmer ointment.
- **Poultice or Fomentation:** Steep or decoct the herbs and wrap them in thin cloth, then bind them to the site of application. A steeping bag may be used to hold the poultice and kept in place with plastic wrap or a cloth bandage.
- **Dosage:** The usual dosage for herb medicine is one or two cups of tea a day. However, all people are not alike. Some are strong, and others are weak; therefore, some require strong tea, while others need a weaker tea. You can determine the proper amount by starting with one cupful a day. If the effect is too strong, reduce; if it is too weak, increase until desired effects are reached. Some herbs are bitter. To compensate, add honey or sugar to taste, or brew it as usual but dilute with warm water, either sweetened or not. For best results, use the tea for three days, then omit for a day or two, and then continue again. Repeat this method until the tea is no longer needed.
- **Use Good Sense:** All of the herbs listed in this book are indicated for medical use, but note that some of them produce unpleasant effects, and therefore you must familiarize yourself with the medical terminology herein. A "cathartic" is not the same as a "laxative," and it is your responsibility to learn and know the difference. If your trouble is of a serious nature, your doctor should be consulted.

TRADITIONAL HERBAL REMEDIES

Once you understand the basic principles of herbology, you will be able to devise your own combinatory recipes, based on your preference for certain herbs and on which herbs are most easily available to you. These simple recipes may serve to get you started. Be sure to check all herbs for side effects before mixing them into your recipes.

ANTHELMINTIC TEA

Caution is requested of those who take vermifuge or anthelmintic teas, as a too-strong dose may carry side effects. Combine any of these: Arbor Vitæ, Wafer Ash, Butternut Bark, Horehound, Lamb's Quarters, Male Fern, Pomegranate, Pumpkin Seed, Southernwood. Wormseed, Wormwood.

BLOOD PURIFIER TEA

A mixture of Bilberry, Red Clover, Thyme, and Strawberry Leaves makes an excellent blood purifier.

CARMINATIVE TEA

Canada Snake Root's carminative properties are measurably increased when used in combination with Sassafras, Cinnamon, and Peppermint. Other traditional carminatives, used singly or in combination, are the seeds of Anise, Caraway, Cardamom, Coriander, Dill, and Fennel, to which candied Ginger can be added as a sweetener.

COUGH AND COLD TEA

Mix two parts Mint, plus one part each Horehound, Hyssop, Lemon Balm, Linden Flowers, and Marshmallow, plus half a part each Sage, Borage, and Thyme. Store in a sealed jar. Use 1 spoonful per cup of hot water to make tea. Sweeten with honey; add a squeeze of Lemon juice and a capful of brandy.

DIURETIC TEA

Diuretics work well in combination. You do not need them all to make an effective tea, but blending a few makes their action more sure: Althæa Leaf, White Ash, Broom Tops, Button Snake Root, Canada Snake Root, Caraway, Chicory Root, Cleavers, Slippery Elm Bark, Figwort, Gravel Root, Horsetail Grass, Juniper Berries, Marshmallow Root, Saxifrage, and Uva-Ursi.

ALTHÆA'S HOT LEMON AND CHICKEN SOUP FOR COLDS

This soup relieves throat troubles and catarrh. To a cup of water, add ¼ teaspoon Chicken Soup Base and ⅛ teaspoon Miso Soybean Paste. Heat on the stove at high. Add ⅛ teaspoon Aji Amarillo Powder (Yellow Hot Pepper Powder), remove from heat, and add the juice and pulp of ½ Lemon. Allow the patient to dilute this with warm water to taste and temperature. For variety, add orzo pasta or leftover cooked rice while the liquids are heating, remove from heat when cooked, and add crumbled Tuna, the Lemon juice, and fresh Basil. Or make it like a combination of Stracciatella alla Romana and Avgolemono, beating one egg with Parmesan cheese, stirring it in, and adding the Lemon and Basil at the end.

COUGH SYRUP

Simmer 1 oz. each of Boneset, Coltsfoot, Slippery Elm, Horehound, Flax seed, and Licorice root in 1 quart of water until the volume is reduced to $^1/_3$, then strain off the extract. Add to it 1 pint of blackstrap molasses and ½ lb. sugar. Simmer until the sugar is dissolved and seal in bottles for future use. This may be taken freely for cases of cough and bronchitis.

WOMEN'S TONIC

Add ½ oz. Chamomile, ½ oz. Sweet Balm, ¼ oz. Cramp Bark, and ¼ oz. Spikenard to 1 quart Port wine. Let sit 24 hours, shake it, and strain. A cordial glass may be taken as needed for female regulation. Alternatively, extract the herbs in 1 pint of Brandy; the dosage is then 1 Tablespoon only.

FIRST AID POULTICE

All of these herbs are vulneraries or antiseptics: Knotweed, Golden Rod, Lady's Mantle, Calendula, Fenugreek, Fleabane, Plantain Leaf, Gobernadora, Thyme, and Yarrow. Combine equal parts of as many as you can obtain. You do not need them all. Mix them and place a nice "pillow" amount in as many small muslin tea bags as the mixture will fill. Store the muslin bags in a sealed glass jar in a dark place. Always carry one bag of this mixture with you in your first aid kit or purse. If you or your family members suffer a scape, bruise, or cut, put the bag into a cup and just cover it with boiling water. Let the herbs steep at least three minutes, allow the tea-liquid to cool, use it to wash the wound, and pack the herb bag on the wound as a poultice. Hold it in place with plastic wrap, a cloth bandage, or duct tape. If you can add fresh-cut garlic to the herb bag at the time of use, do so, as it too is antiseptic.

HEALING SKIN SALVE

For chapped skin, hemorrhoids, and sore udders of Goats and Cows, melt 1 cup lard or tallow, add to it ¼ cup petroleum jelly and/or ⅛ cup beeswax, then put into it, until it will hold no more, equal parts of as many of these herbs as you can get: Yellow Dock, Marshmallow roots or leaves, Celandine, and Comfrey root or leaves. Keep on the fire until the lard mixture is a dark green, then strain through cheesecloth into a coloured glass jar and close it up. When hardened, apply freely to the affected area twice a day.

HERPETIC POULTICE

A poultice of equal parts of Celandine, Poke, White Oak, Willow Bark, and Beech Drops is very useful in herpetic affections.

A WELL-REGARDED HAIR TONIC

Peppergrass, Cedarwood, Rosemary, Thyme, Lavender, Sage, and Bay are said to stimulate the scalp and give vitality to the hair. Prepare them as an infusion and pour the liquid over the head, then wrap the hair in a towel that has been thoroughly wetted with the same liquid. Remove when the towel cools. The infusion can also be mixed into your regular shampoo.

To make this up as an oil-based tonic, you will need the essential oil of each of these herbs except Peppergrass, plus Vitamin E oil and any type of vegetable oil as a base. Since Peppergrass is not available as an essential oil, start by making infused Peppergrass oil. Pack dried Peppergrass in your carrier oil, gently heat it for an hour, allow it to cool, strain the oil, and repeat for a total of three "runs" of Peppergrass. For every 4 oz. of infused oil, add 8 drops of each of the essential oils, plus 8 drops of Vitamin E oil.

MOTH REPELLENT SACHET FOR WOOLENS

Patchouli, Wormwood, Tansy, Lavender, Rosemary, Cedar shavings, and Cloves mixed together in equal parts and sewn into in loosely-woven cloth sachets will make an excellent moth repellent for woolens.

PLEASING SACHET FOR LINENS

Caraway, Cinnamon, Cloves, Mace, Nutmeg, and Tonka Beans make a fragrant sachet for linens. Grind the ingredients coarsely and put into loosely-woven cloth sachets. This mixture is far more pleasing than the Moth Repellent Sachet above, but it is not as preservative of woolen goods.

BIBLIOGRAPHY

Balch, Phyllis A. *Prescription for Herbal Healing,* Avery Trade 2002.

Bremness, Lesley. *Herbs (Eyewitness Handbooks).* Dorling Kindersley, 1994.

Brown, Deni. *The Herb Society of America Encyclopedia of Herbs and Their Uses.* Dorling Kindersley, 1995.

Cook, Wm. H. *The Physiomedical Dispensatory, a Treatise on Therapeutics, Materia Medica, and Pharmacy in Accordance with the Principles of Physiological Medication.* Wm. H. Cook, 1869.

Culpeper, Nicholas. *The English Physician*, also published as *The Complete Herbal.* 1652 (and many subsequent enlarged, revised, corrected, and abridged editions.

de Waal, Marinus. *Medicines From The Bible.* translated by Jane Meijlink-Green. Samuel Weiser, 1994. [Original Dutch publication by Uitgeverij Schors, 1980.]

Gerad, John. *Gerard's Herball, Or, Generall Historie of Plantes.* John Norton, 1597 (and many subsequent enlarged, revised, corrected, and abridged editions).

Grieve, Mrs. M[aude]. *A Modern Herbal.* Jonathan Cape, 1931. Reprinted in facsimile, Dover Publications, 1982.

Hoffmann, David. *Holistic Herbal: A Safe and Practical Guide to Making and Using Herbal Remedies.* Thorsons, 2003.

Hutchens, Alma R. *Indian Herbology of North America.* Merco, 1969. Reprinted by Shamballa, 1991.

King, John, with Harvey Wickes Felter and John Uri Lloyd. *King's American Dispensatory.* 3rd revised edition. Ohio Valley Co., 1898.

Kress, Henriette. *Practical Herbs.* Yrtit ja Yrttiterapia, 2013.

Mathews, F. Schuyler. *Field Book of American Wildflowers.* Knickerbocker Press, 1902; New Edition Revised and Enlarged, G. P. Putnam's Sons, 1912.

Meyer, Clarence. *The Herbalist Almanac: A Fifty Year Anthology.* Meyerbooks, 1988.

Meyer, Joseph E. *The Herbalist.* Revised and enlarged by Clarence Meyer; additional material by David C. Meyer. Meyerbooks, many editions, 1918-1981.

Millspaugh, Charles F. *Medicinal Plants, an Illustrated and Descriptive Guide to Plants Indigenous to and Naturalized in the United States Which Are Used in Medicine.* John C. Yorston and Co., 1892. Reprinted as *American Medicinal Plants.* Dover Publications, 1974.

Nickell, J. M. *J. M. Nickell's Botanical Ready Reference, Especially Designed for Druggists and Physicians, Containing All of the Botanical Drugs Known Up to the Present Time, Giving Their Medical Properties and All of Their Botanical, Common, Pharmacopœial and German Common (in German) Names.* J. M. Nickell, 1881. Reprinted in facsimile, Trinity Center Press, 1976.

Porter, Gene Stratton. *The Harvester.* Doubleday, Page & Co., 1911.

Rickett, Harold William. *The New Field Book of American Wildflowers.* G. P. Putnam's Sons, 1963.